PROFESSOR PETER TYRER is a community psychiatrist engaged in outreach and rehabilitation in Paddington and also Head of the Department of Psychological Medicine at Imperial College, London. He has a range of qualifications including Fellowship of the Academy of Medical Sciences. He has been engaged in stress research and related areas, particularly tranquillizer dependence and personality problems, since 1970, and is on the editorial board of several journals, including *Stress and Health*. He takes his work seriously, but is less stringent with himself and has a quirky sense of humour, aggravated by the existence of an exact double – an identical twin, who is also a psychiatrist – and by working as gardener to Spike Milligan many years ago. He still retains a close interest in gardening, living close to one of the horticultural gems of London, Kew Gardens, and aims to combine his botanical and psychiatric interests with, fortunately rare, recourse to herbal remedies.

Overcoming Common Problems Series

A full list of titles is available from Sheldon Press,
1 Marylebone Road, London NW1 4DU, and on our website at
www.sheldonpress.co.uk

Overcoming Common Problems Series

Coping with Stammering
Trudy Stewart and Jackie Turnbull

Coping with Stomach Ulcers
Dr Tom Smith

Coping with Strokes
Dr Tom Smith

Coping with Suicide
Maggie Helen

Coping with Thrush
Caroline Clayton

Coping with Thyroid Problems
Dr Joan Gomez

Curing Arthritis – The Drug-Free Way
Margaret Hills

Curing Arthritis – More Ways to a
Drug-Free Life
Margaret Hills

Curing Arthritis Diet Book
Margaret Hills

Curing Arthritis Exercise Book
Margaret Hills and Janet Horwood

Cystic Fibrosis – A Family Affair
Jane Chumbley

Depression at Work
Vicky Maud

Depressive Illness
Dr Tim Cantopher

Fertility
Julie Reid

The Fibromyalgia Healing Diet
Christine Craggs-Hinton

Garlic
Karen Evennett

Getting a Good Night's Sleep
Fiona Johnston

The Good Stress Guide
Mary Hartley

Heal the Hurt: How to Forgive and Move
On
Dr Ann Macaskill

Heart Attacks – Prevent and Survive
Dr Tom Smith

Helping Children Cope with Attention
Deficit Disorder
Dr Patricia Gilbert

Helping Children Cope with Bullying
Sarah Lawson

Helping Children Cope with Divorce
Rosemary Wells

Helping Children Cope with Grief
Rosemary Wells

Helping Children Cope with Stammering
Jackie Turnbull and Trudy Stewart

Helping Children Get the Most from School
Sarah Lawson

How to Accept Yourself
Dr Windy Dryden

How to Be Your Own Best Friend
Dr Paul Hauck

How to Cope when the Going Gets Tough
Dr Windy Dryden and Jack Gordon

How to Cope with Anaemia
Dr Joan Gomez

How to Cope with Bulimia
Dr Joan Gomez

How to Cope with Difficult People
Alan Houel with Christian Godefroy

How to Cope with Stress
Dr Peter Tyrer

How to Enjoy Your Retirement
Vicky Maud

How to Get Where You Want to Be
Christian Godefroy

How to Improve Your Confidence
Dr Kenneth Hambly

How to Keep Your Cholesterol in Check
Dr Robert Povey

How to Lose Weight Without Dieting
Mark Barker

How to Love and Be Loved
Dr Paul Hauck

How to Make Yourself Miserable
Dr Windy Dryden

How to Pass Your Driving Test
Donald Ridland

How to Raise Confident Children
Carole Baldock

How to Stand up for Yourself
Dr Paul Hauck

How to Stick to a Diet
Deborah Steinberg and Dr Windy Dryden

How to Stop Worrying
Dr Frank Tallis

The How to Study Book
Alan Brown

Overcoming Common Problems Series

Overcoming Common Problems

How to Cope with Stress

Professor Peter Tyrer
MD, FRCP, FRCPsych, FFPHM, FMedSci

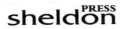

To Mark and Beryl
for helping with mine

First published in Great Britain in 1980 by
Sheldon Press
1 Marylebone Road
London NW1 4DU

New edition 2003

British Library Cataloguing-in-Publication Data
A catalogue record for this book is available from the British Library

ISBN 0–85969–880–7

1 3 5 7 9 10 8 6 4 2

Typeset by Deltatype Ltd, Birkenhead, Wirral
Printed in Great Britain by Biddles Ltd
www.biddles.co.uk

Contents

Acknowledgements

Revising books can sometimes be a chore and involve much undervalued effort. I thank Linda Coachworth and Michelle Clark for making the task easier and preventing too many foolish flights of fancy.

Introduction

When we talk to our friends, pick up a newspaper, listen to the radio or watch television, we are bound to hear or see stress mentioned over and over again. Perhaps we hear it so often that it ceases to have any impact. A visitor from another planet coming across the word for the first time would have great difficulty in knowing what stress is, where it comes from and goes to, and how it is caused. From birth to death we seem to be surrounded by stress. A mother becomes moody and depressed after childbirth; the stress of a difficult birth is blamed. The baby frequently cries and keeps the family awake at night. The father loses his temper and batters the child. Later, in court, the stress of coping with a new baby is blamed. He gets upset by the court appearance, gets headaches and feelings of tension and has a great deal of time off work. Stress is blamed again. Meanwhile, his mother is convicted for shoplifting. She has never done this before and her defence is that the stress of the onset of menopause made her act completely out of character. Soon after this her husband dies. He had only just been retired by his firm and his early death is blamed on the stress of being 'put on the scrapheap' before his time. His death provokes repercussions in his family and his wife becomes depressed because she cannot accept that he has gone. So the round of stress goes on like a macabre dance. To cap it all, our planetary visitor will learn that, as we now live in a 'stressful society', there is no way in which we can avoid stress; like time, it affects us all in the same way.

Our alien could draw several conclusions from these observations of us. First, stress is everywhere and, as it seems to be a recent phenomenon, it is probably a mysterious virus or bacterium that infects us from birth. Second, stress is unpleasant and apparently has little to do with happy events. Third, stress is somehow related to change. If the alien was a cynical observer it might reject all these conclusions and decide that stress does not really exist but is merely a scapegoat. When anything goes wrong in the lives of these strange humans the magical word 'stress' is invoked as the universal excuse. Our visitor would also be surprised at the way in which we go about coping with and preventing stress. Businesspeople who become stressed by sitting in offices in polluted cities making executive decisions are encouraged to take healthy exercise whenever possible, yet young people, who may spend a large part of their time exercising, are put under pressure to improve their status by gaining qualifications that involve spending long periods doing sedentary work. If they are 'successful', they may eventually reach a position where they can sit in offices all day making executive decisions and being stressed, one of the perks of the job being membership of a health club!

In trying to solve such curious paradoxes, our visitor would be puzzled further by the tremendous differences in people's ideas of stress. While some will never take a journey by aeroplane because they find even the thought of flying too stressful to contemplate, others, who look and appear to be from exactly the same species, take up hang-gliding as a hobby, considering it pleasant and exciting to fly through the air on an unpredictable course decided by the elements so that the place of landing is quite uncertain. Some are so concerned about traffic that they will not cross a busy street – a decision our visitor would probably regard as sensible after seeing our roads. Yet, our alien would also observe that motor racing is a popular sport and it depends on forcing dangerous vehicles to the limits of speed and endurance round sharp bends that increase the risk of damage to driver and car and, what is more, people pay to watch it because they find it pleasurable.

After our visitor has rubbed its eyes and scratched its head in disbelief at the illogical behaviour of these stress-ridden Earthlings, it might hope to be enlightened by looking at medical ways of treating stress. By now the alien would be quite certain that stress is a disease, for nothing healthy could cause people to behave in this way. At least our visitor would find some consistency in this area, but it would still be difficult to relate to the ideas about stress that it came across earlier.

Stress is reduced by techniques that involve slowing down rather than speeding up. The slowing down can be achieved in many ways – talking to people, taking prescribed medicines, learning to relax, doing special exercises, such as in yoga and meditation, having a holiday or just taking it easy for a few days. As much of human behaviour is geared to speeding up rather than slowing down, our visitor might be surprised, but by now it would probably have become used to the inconsistencies of this strange species. After surveying the range of treatments available for stress, it could hardly be impressed by them. After all, if they are really effective, why is everyone still complaining about stress and its effects? Our alien's scepticism would be increased if it looked at the large number of books and papers written about stress and its 'correct' treatment. After returning to its spaceship, there would be only one way of describing what it had heard and seen without being accused of making everything up. The population of planet Earth is masochistic. Earthlings make their lives unpleasant and then complain about it, but they really enjoy this discomfort because all their efforts are designed to make it worse. They call this consequence of their errors 'stress' because they are afraid to admit that they are the real culprits.

Before you dismiss this conclusion as fanciful, read on. This book is published as part of the 'Overcoming Common Problems' series, but overcoming stress is not a realistic aim, although many set out to achieve it. In any case, stress has its good points as well as its bad ones and life without stress is not life, but death. Stress is not always something outside ourselves for which we can point the finger of blame at others. It often comes from inside and, although we can often point to people, events and places as having a part to play in our reactions, they are not the only causes. We do not have to be the prisoners of our surroundings and, to live with stress effectively, we must either change our circumstances or ourselves. This is not an easy task and many of us find it easier to blame someone or something else beyond our control. Grumbling in this way will not help anyone, apart from a minority who genuinely like to grumble – it can be a form of stress relief – and suffering will go on if nothing else is done to alter the situation.

Even if you feel that there is nothing that can be done for your stress problems you may find something of value in this book, which emphasizes coping, not conquering. I do not promise any instant cures and you may be annoyed at some of the things I say along the way, but, stay with me and think whether or not any of the advice I give might have a bearing on difficulties you are having now or have had in the past. Throughout this book I will be emphasizing that stress is a highly individual reaction and so solutions to it have to be specially tailored. So, although some of the advice I give may seem like complete nonsense, there should be some that really strikes home and leads to corrective action.

This is the second edition of a book that was first published in 1980. In revising it, I have been surprised at how little the main message has changed in the last 23 years, even though our knowledge is considerably greater. Although we know much more, we are not very good at putting it to positive effect. Perhaps when you have read this book you will understand why. It is more about adjustments than finding solutions.

1

What is stress?

People learning English often complain that, although it is easy to pick up at first, it is very difficult to learn properly because the words have so many different meanings. Indeed, one of my German colleagues goes one step further, saying that English is a deceitful language because you never know where you are with it and it can strike back and humiliate you just when you think you have it conquered. The word 'stress' is a good example of this problem. First of all, it is a grammatical anarchist. It breaks all the rules and behaves as a noun, verb and adjective, whenever it so pleases.

This is illustrated by a sentence recently spoken by one of my psychologist colleagues after seeing someone who, in ordinary lay language, was suffering from a stress illness. He was being questioned about the diagnosis – the technical label that is used to classify illnesses – and some people were questioning whether or not the diagnosis was more typical of a depressive illness. He replied, 'I stress the word stress as stress is the most distressing aspect of her symptoms – a direct response to losing her job – that is why I regard it as an acute stress reaction rather than a depressive problem.' Here we have the word stress used four times – twice as a noun, once as a verb and once as an adjective. It is immediately understandable to an English person but not always to others, and it is not hard to see why. It is difficult to think of any other word that could replace 'stress' each time in this sentence and still make grammatical sense.

The problem is that stress as a word comes from two sources. The first is the feeling of strain, of tension, with stress really representing a shorter form of 'distress'. This is perhaps the common understanding of stress as meant in the title of this book – the idea that an external force (or sometimes an internal one) is acting on the person and creating pressure. Interestingly, this is also the meaning of the word in physics, where stress and strain can be defined quite precisely. The second meaning of stress is emphasis – both as a noun, in the sense of to lay stress on a subject or word or event, and as a verb, 'I want to stress that . . .', as in the psychologist's words above.

Although the second meaning is different from the first, it overlaps more than appears at first sight. Thus David Crystal, the author of *The Cambridge Encyclopaedia of the English Language* (Cambridge University Press, 1995), in writing about the significance of stress or intonation of a word, illustrates the point by describing nine ways of saying 'yes' to the highly significant question – sometimes the most significant question in a person's life – 'Will you marry me?'

Nine ways, you may ask? How can you answer yes in nine ways? Well, you can. Depending on the stress, or intonation, given to each part of this single syllable, the answer can vary in presentation from surprise – 'I never expected this' – to boredom – 'here we go again' – to puzzlement – 'do you really know what you are saying?' – to suspicion – 'what's the catch?' – to quiet acceptance – 'I've been prepared for this' – to indifference – 'I'm thinking about it, but only thinking' – to shock – 'I'm completely pole-axed' – to doubt – 'I'm agreeing but there are a lot of problems ahead' – and to excited haste – 'I can't wait to get to the altar in case you change your mind'. Try practising some of these and you will learn why breach of promise is so difficult to prove and why James Joyce considered 'yes' to be the most powerful word in the English language and why 'yeah' is such a powerful part of songs by the Beatles.

So we can conclude that stress is concerned with emphasis and pressure, and implicit in this is the idea that it disturbs the equilibrium of life. This loss of equilibrium need not cause problems, but, when we consider the other meaning of stress, distress, it is common to assume that all stress must be unpleasant. However, this is where I part company with this common assumption. A stress need not be unpleasant; some people even seek it out. Most people who read this book will not be impressed by the positive value of stress, and, after all, the title, *How to Cope with Stress* implies that it is something to be avoided. However, it is important not to forget the positive aspects. You will be reminded of them again.

Stress in action

At this stage, let us look at some examples of stress in action to see if there are any common features that will help us to find a satisfactory definition. All of them are taken from real life and it may help if we consider how we would feel if put through the same experiences.

A young man joins the Navy towards the end of World War II. He is sent out to the Far East and sees action in a battleship in the final year of the war against Japan. His job is to transfer ammunition from the hold to the guns above. The part of the hold where he works is open to the sky and explosives surround him on all sides. Above, Japanese kamikaze pilots weave their way through the barrage of anti-aircraft fire, looking for the chance to plunge to the decks in their human bombs to complete their suicide missions. The young man sees these planes and is reminded over and over again what will happen if a direct hit is scored on his ship. He cannot do anything to prevent it and relies entirely on the accuracy of his fellow gunners. After six months of nerve-racking action he goes to pieces. He rarely sleeps but when he does he has nightmares of air attacks ending in a ball of flame, when he wakes, sweating and terrified. He cannot concentrate and becomes inefficient at his job. He feels weak and has a series of symptoms, headaches, nausea, lack of appetite, loss of weight, nervous twitchings and blurring of vision. He is seen by a medical officer and sent back to England for shore duty.

Compare this stressful experience with that of a young woman. She comes from a staid family who lay great emphasis on accuracy, reliability and security. She has no idea what to do when she leaves school but is persuaded by her parents to become a civil servant as this job requires all the qualities they hold most dear. In the absence of any alternative, she reluctantly agrees and takes up a job as an assistant in a tax office – a job with excellent prospects, a clear promotion ladder and a secure income until retirement age. At first, she works as a ledger clerk checking figures. The others in her office are older than her, but they are polite, well-spoken and helpful. She does her job well and is promoted to senior ledger clerk, now checking the figures of more important financial transactions. She continues to work with kind and considerate colleagues and her parents congratulate themselves on setting her forth on a worthwhile career. However, after six months, she is utterly bored with the apparent triviality of this job. She feels tyrannized by rows of meaningless figures and irritated because they all have to balance on her ledger sheets. She has curious impulses to upset the balance and falsify the figures, impulses to which she eventually succumbs. She sees her superior, hoping to be sacked, but is promoted instead. The pattern of boring, repetitive work among sympathetic, stolid people continues. At last she can stand it no longer. She gives up her job and becomes a sales rep. Her parents are predictably horrified.

Finally, let us look at the case of a long-distance lorry driver who likes his job. It offers him variety and a degree of independence that he would not find elsewhere. True, at times, he feels angry with other drivers on the road who seem not to appreciate the difficulties of driving a ten-ton lorry, but usually he enjoys sitting high above the road with so much throbbing power beneath him. He often prefers to drive for many hours at a stretch, although this means irregular meals and he knows it is frowned on by the company. After several years of continual long-distance driving, he starts to experience pains in his stomach. They often wake him at night and trouble him during long drives. He finds milk drinks helpful and often takes them when he has the pain, but the pain gradually worsens. He goes to see his doctor, who arranges for tests and referral to a specialist in hospital. The tests show that he has a duodenal ulcer. He discusses his future with the specialist and his own doctor and is advised to change his job as long-distance lorry driving is thought to be too stressful for him.

The core elements of stress

In all three situations, the problems have been caused by stress, but it is very difficult to find a common pattern in them. Most of us would sympathize strongly with the first man as he had been through a highly unpleasant experience, one in which he had lost all power to control the most threatening dangers he was facing. Although most of us can tolerate the same degree of danger for short periods, it becomes more difficult the longer it goes on and, sooner or later, we all crack up.

The second example is more puzzling. Those of us who have tidy, methodical minds and prefer an organized routine in life would find it hard to understand why the young woman should have reacted so strangely. Those who like more excitement in their lives and would not contemplate a career in the civil service would understand her reaction only too well and would be surprised that she lasted as long as six months in the job.

Our third example also provokes different feelings. Those of us who have never had serious indigestion or stomach pains would see him as a man with a satisfying job who just happened to develop a duodenal ulcer. Of course we may have read somewhere that duodenal ulcers are caused by stress, but this would mean little to us unless we too had experienced indigestion when under stress. Then we would appreciate his symptoms only too well and probably would relieve them in similar ways.

The only common feature is conflict. This takes a mental form in the first two cases and a physical form in the third. For some reason they and their surroundings do not mix properly and they cannot adapt in a healthy way. Beyond that, they disagree. The common view of stress is as something that puts us under increased pressure and forces us to act and think more quickly or intensely than we would like. However, our tax clerk in her quiet office leisurely looking at figures is not under this kind of pressure. It is probably less than she would like. She finds it stressful because part of her shouts stridently through the conventional façade, 'Get me out of here, this isn't me!' This brings up one of the most important points about stress.

Stress is not defined by its cause but by a person's reaction to this cause – technically called the 'stressor'.

Stress can be positive or negative

Those of us who could not tolerate being in the civil service and have duodenal ulcers would probably see all three of the situations just described as stressful. By contrast, a healthy tax-collector who actually likes the job and enjoys parachute jumping in any spare time (such people do exist) would find none of them stressful, although even such a person would find it difficult to remain settled in the battleship at war. This is why predicting stress is such a problem. It is easy to look back on an experience, knowing it has done harm and say that it was the stress of X or Y that caused it. It is quite another matter to predict in advance that someone is likely to be harmed by going through a particular experience. The precision and the power of the high-quality retrospectoscope are immense, but it is all part of the scientific superstructure of being clever afterwards. The reasons we are often wrong when we try to predict stressful reactions is that human beings, these amazing creatures described so accurately by Shakespeare as 'how noble in reason, how infinite in faculties, in form and moving how express and admirable, in action, how like an angel, in apprehension, how like a god', are also 'in adaptation, how like a chameleon'. We can turn the most unpleasant experiences and environments to our advantage or suffer them for intolerable lengths of time supported only by hope.

5

So the effects of stress may be positive or negative, and they can affect both the mind and the body. A common fallacy about stress is that it is essentially a nervous reaction. Our third example would not be included if this were true, because the first sign of stress that he experienced was the pain of his duodenal ulcer. Now, if we had the key to his mind and could recall everything that he had been through over the years, we would find that all was not as well as he made out and his lifestyle was in fact a stressful one. However, the mind has a great ability to cast unwelcome feelings aside if they disagree with others that are strongly held. Our lorry driver could not be accused of dishonesty when he said he liked his job and found it satisfying. However, the mind and body are closely intertwined and stress can show itself in the body's reactions without the conscious mind being aware that anything is up.

Defining stress

The best definition of the special form of stress described in this book is that it is *the reaction of the mind and body to change*. This covers all the examples of stress that we have described and a great deal more. You will find other definitions of stress elsewhere and I do not pretend that this is the right one. My definition is very broad and takes in a large range of reactions that many people do not find unpleasant even though they involve a great deal of change. The key issue is whether or not we adapt to the change when it takes place. If we do, the stress is hardly noticed; if we do not, the stress becomes distress. It persists and may eventually create mental and physical ill health.

The definition includes all kinds of change – pleasant, unpleasant, exciting and boring. The stress of winning a fortune on the football pools can lead to distress in time if we do not adjust to it, and adjustment is often not as easy as we might think. If we do not adapt to the initial change, distress will go on continuously in the absence of further variation, but change always sets off the process. People react differently to change because they have different personalities and different ways of coping. Some situations are so unpleasant that the initial stress always moves on to distress. The situation of the young man on the battleship described earlier is so threatening that very few people could adapt to it completely, but that of working in a tax office involves only a slight change from normal for most people. Only a small number would find that they could not adapt to this and so become distressed. So when we say that something or other is stressful, we really mean that the change it produces is large and most people would find difficulty in adjusting to it. We cannot say that *all* people, without exception, would become distressed.

At the other end of the scale are changes that appear so small we cannot see any possible problems in adapting, but they will loom much larger in the thinking of some people who cannot adjust easily. Each personality is different and we all have at least one weak spot, an Achilles heel that can cause all sorts of problems.

We cannot alter people's basic personalities, although experience and age may change them quite considerably (see the Further reading list at the end of the book). In coming to terms with stress, we try to adjust as well as possible to all the changes going on about us. Many of these adjustments take place without our knowing much about them, but some bother us continually. The latter are the ones that make us feel 'under stress', force us to seek advice or take other forms of action to remove them. If we could always adjust to stress, we should never become distressed.

What makes some suffer from stress and others take it in their stride? Before answering this we need to know what goes on in our minds and bodies when we are under stress, and to decide when the stress is helpful and when it is harmful.

2

How stress affects your mind and body

Think of the time you last had to run to catch a train or bus or, indeed, took any vigorous exercise. If you have not done these things, just remember looking at athletes on television or in a film, particularly in short sprint races. You will have noticed a host of feelings, expressions and behaviours, most of which you are seldom aware of when you are relaxed.

Breathing becomes deeper and quicker. This is shown on the outside by puffing and blowing as more air is forced in and out of the chest as though someone inside was operating a hidden bellows. You are likely to be aware of your heart beating – I mean beating with an insistence that cannot be ignored, forcing itself to be noticed. Under normal circumstances, it ticks over without any bother to your consciousness. As well as feeling it hammering away in your chest, you may also experience pulsating feelings in your neck, as though streams of contractions were passing from your heart along the blood vessels. Your muscles will be tense and active even if they are not involved in your athletic movements. This is best seen in your face, which is stretched into peculiar shapes by tension in its muscles, the agony of effort. If it is a hot day, you will sweat soon after the exercise begins. At first the sweating will be confined to your palms, soles of your feet, armpits and face, but then, as you get hotter, beads of perspiration will spring up all over the surface of your body. On the other hand, your mouth will feel steadily drier the longer you are active, with eventually your tongue feeling like coarse sandpaper in a hot kiln.

All these feelings are caused by your body trying to respond to the extra demands you are making, yet at the same time compensating for these demands so that internal change is kept to a minimum. When you are physically active, your muscles are working harder and need more oxygen from your blood. Automatic mechanisms (reflexes) come into play so that the heart pumps harder and quicker, and more of the blood is diverted to the muscles where all the extra work is being done. However, the amount of blood in your body does not alter, so, if more goes to the muscles, less has to go elsewhere. It is the skin, intestines and other digestive organs that receive less. This is the main reason for your mouth feeling dry when you are very active and why, at the beginning before your body has heated up, the skin is pale. The glands that keep the mouth moist with saliva are not just there to keep the mouth wet, but are also part of the digestive organs. When they receive less blood, they become less active and your mouth is no longer well lubricated. Meanwhile, your muscles work away and burn up most of the oxygen from your blood and replace it with carbon dioxide. When the level of carbon dioxide in the bloodstream rises, your breathing is stimulated, so you puff and blow. This gets rid of the extra carbon dioxide and also takes more oxygen into the blood, which is pumped to the muscles. So each of the demands you set in motion by your energies is followed by your body, but only at the cost of less activity elsewhere. You temporarily throw your body off balance by your dramatic changes, but it quickly catches up. You will notice that it does not catch up completely as, when you stop exercising, it takes a few minutes for your sweating to stop, your muscles to relax and your heartbeat and breathing to return to normal. The fitter you are, the shorter this time will be.

If you compare these feelings with those experienced at a time when you felt emotionally keyed up in any way – angry, anxious, excited or frightened – you will recognize many similarities. You breathe more deeply and quickly, your heart pumps faster, your face, palms and soles of your feet sweat (but there is little elsewhere) and your muscles feel tense. The difference is that you are not usually physically energetic at such times. All these changes can go on without you moving from your chair – they are all part of preparation for action. Your body receives impulses from your mind saying, 'I realize that you are a bit slow on the uptake, so I'm giving you ample warning that I'm liable to swing into emergency action in the very near future!' So the body primes its emergency systems and anticipates action even if it never happens. Physical and emotional stress are essentially the same, except that emotional stress seldom reaches the same intensity in its demands on the body. It is also worth remembering that the body does not take any notice of the kind of emotion being shown. It makes no difference whether you are red in the face from anger or hot and bothered with embarrassment, the body reacts in the same way.

What is going on?
An introduction to the autonomic nervous system

These healthy reactions of the body to stress are mainly controlled by a special part of the nervous system called the 'autonomic nervous system'. 'Autonomic' means self-governing, and the name illustrates that the system organizes itself without any interference from outside. There are two parts to the system that normally remain in balance. The 'sympathetic' part is the one that gears you for action and makes you aware of your body functioning. It is sometimes called the 'fight or flight' response because most emergencies involve running away from a danger or advancing towards conflict. It can be brought into operation fairly quickly because, in addition to nervous stimulation, there are hormones secreted into the blood at such times that rapidly pass round the body and stimulate the organs for action. The chief hormone is adrenaline, which stimulates the heart and muscles and makes you aware of its effects in only a few seconds.

For balance, we have the 'parasympathetic system'. Its job is best summed up by the phrase 'rest and digest'. When you are most calm outwardly your parasympathetic system is at its most energetic. It is responsible for rest and sleep, organizing the digestion and breakdown of food, storing up supplies in the body ready for use in an emergency and keeping everything ticking over nicely. It takes much longer to come into operation than the sympathetic system and works at its best when there is least interruption, which is usually when you are asleep.

If you think of a country at war and then compare what it is like in peacetime, you get a good idea of the two different systems. The declaration of war is an emergency and mobilization is urgent. As quickly as possible, factories have to be converted from the needs of peace to those of war. Thus, the production of cars, washing machines, refrigerators and farm machinery is cut down and replaced by that of tanks, guns, armoured cars, missiles and aircraft and, in the world after the events of September 11th 2001, intelligence gathering. People are transferred from their jobs to the armed services and most of the country's budget goes into the war effort.

In peacetime, the priorities are different. People are concerned with achieving a higher standard of living and making their lives more comfortable, so many more goods to achieve these ends are made for them to buy.

Apart from the obvious differences in activity between the two systems, you will probably have noticed another. The peacetime system is much more balanced than the wartime one. That is why you hear so much fuss about the balance of payments. If a country at peace cannot balance what it sells and buys from abroad, its economy runs into trouble. A country on a war footing is different. It is almost expected to be out of balance, to run up debts that will be paid off after the war, which is why post-war credits, war bonds and other arrangements for paying for the war become necessary. The policy becomes 'let us put everything into the fight so we can win as quickly as possible', even if this means being in hock for years afterwards. When the war is over, the balancing peacetime system has to pay off these debts as well as try to satisfy the demand for improved living standards.

Likewise, the sympathetic system puts the body temporarily out of balance when it comes into operation and the parasympathetic system has to make up for it afterwards. The activity of the sympathetic system is part of healthy stress when it is only temporary and can soon be corrected. If the sympathetic stimulation goes on for too long unopposed by the parasympathetic, however, it becomes impossible to get compensation afterwards and the stress is no longer healthy.

The key difference between healthy and harmful stress is that in healthy stress there is rapid adjustment to the change and in harmful stress there is little or no adjustment. This point is critical to understanding and coping with stress. Remember our definition of stress – the reaction of mind and body to change. We are surrounded by changes and have no trouble in adjusting to most of them. It is only those changes that we have no answer to that lead to harmful stress, the sort of stress that people complain about and causes physical and mental suffering. Let us see how uncompensated stress can do harm.

The adaptation syndrome

Remember the man with the duodenal ulcer that we came across in the last chapter. He was not consciously aware of his fight or flight response coming into action while he was driving his lorry. This is because the stimulation of his sympathetic nervous system was only a mild one, but it persisted. When this happens, the body has another

11

little trick. Another group of hormones – the main one being cortisone – is secreted into the blood and sets the body's defences at a higher level so it can withstand the stress. However, this cannot go on indefinitely and sooner or later these defences fail.

One of the foremost experts on stress, Dr Hans Selye, whose own definition of stress is 'the non-specific result of any demand on the body', first described the effects of stress on the body in 1936 and described it as the 'adaptation syndrome'. This is shown in three parts. The first (alarm) stage is the initial response of fight or flight (operated via the sympathetic nervous system). The second stage is that of resistance, which comes about if the stress continues. This is the time that the body is only able to adapt by great efforts to compensate and this throws a strain on the body's defences. The third stage is exhaustion. The body, or part of it, gives up the fight and dies.

Again, it is useful to think of this process as being similar to a country at war. When war is declared, the mobilization that follows is rapid and responsive to the threat. If the enemy focuses its attack heavily in one place, the defences are often only able to hold firm by diverting resources from elsewhere, thereby making the country more vulnerable to attack from another quarter. If this fails, defeat follows. Of course, the defeat may be a minor one followed by regrouping and regaining of the lost territory, but it can also consist of complete surrender.

So it is with the body and mind when they are faced with stress. There is constant activity, reorganization of resources, surprise attacks and heroic defences, rearguard actions and wild forays, and we are only aware of a small proportion of these on the surface.

Which parts of the body are damaged or die vary from person to person and also depend on the type of stress experienced. It would be wrong to think of our lorry driver's duodenal ulcer being caused only by the stress of driving long distances. One other stress is the irregular hours of work. If you work for 16 hours a day, your parasympathetic system does not get enough time to do its work. A second is irregular meals, often of the wrong sorts of food. A combination of these three stresses picks out the duodenum – the part of the intestine just below the stomach – as the weakest link in the body's chain of defences. The cells on its surface die and the acid from the stomach juices burns a hole in the lining. For the ulcer to heal, the parasympathetic nervous system needs plenty of time to bring the stomach and intestine back into balance. A combination of regular meals of bland foods, changing to a more settled job and increased periods of relaxation are needed. Of course, the ulcer can also be helped by taking medicines or having surgery, but it is likely to recur if other adjustments to lifestyle are not made as well.

Stress and the body

Mental (or emotional) stress may not be involved at all. For example, the physical stress of being overweight can cause a great deal of damage on its own. If you are 63.5 kg (10 stone) overweight, your bones and joints have to work much harder in supporting and transporting the extra load, a load they are not equipped to cope with indefinitely. After resisting valiantly for years, the linings of the joints would wear out. The roughened surfaces would then rub together, producing the pain and swelling of arthritis. If you told an overweight person with arthritis that he was suffering from stress, he would probably be highly indignant. It is a stereotype but is quite often the case that fat people are usually placid and, as stress implies 'nerves', he would deny any connection. However, stress is stress whatever its source and the body does not differentiate.

This does not mean that all bodily disease is due to, or provoked by, stress. Many conditions, such as diabetes, pass down from one generation to another and there is very little we can do to prevent them (although genetic advances may change this situation dramatically). Some diseases, however, even if they seem to come right out of the blue, are caused by stress that has been ignored, dismissed or denied. Detection is the first sign of recognition and can be a great help in finding solutions, as sometimes we do everything possible to avoid detection of stress. Alcohol, discussed later in this book, is commonly turned to to relieve stress, but it is also a stress creator when used to excess. Put simply, alcohol is a poison if given in sufficient quantity, but, because it has pleasurable effects (or continuing to drink prevents unpleasurable ones, such as withdrawal symptoms), many who are hooked on this dangerous, but socially approved, drug pretend there is nothing wrong when it is clear to everybody else that their drinking is creating problem after problem.

I hope that you will have a good idea if you or others in your life are ignoring damaging stress by the time you finish this book, but I doubt it. It often takes a lot of thinking to change and all I can hope to do is set the process, or some doubts, in motion. At the opposite extreme, it would be wrong to blame stress for all illnesses that we cannot understand. In the Middle Ages, when only very little was known about the natural world, anything unexplained was put down to divine intervention (the God of the Gaps). 'Man proposes but God disposes', were the famous words of Thomas à Kempis in the fourteenth century. A paraphrase might be, 'man can pretend to be in charge, but, in the last resort, God is in control and will decide'. In modern society, where religious influences are less prominent than they used to be, there is a danger that stress will take over from God as the universal explanation for the inexplicable, that 'the God of the Gaps' will be replaced by 'Stress fills the Gaps'. This would be wrong, because, to go back to Hans Selye's original definition of stress, it is the 'non-specific' result of a demand on the body and non-specific in this context means 'common' or 'general'. If there is a disease waiting to be discovered that has a 'specific' cause, it is not a consequence of stress. We must not cease to enquire, prematurely concluding that some form of stress is the cause.

This is not to say that stress cannot contribute to disease even when there is a known cause. Take high blood pressure, for example. In emergencies, the sympathetic nervous system stimulates the heart and circulation and in emotional and physical stress the extra work may cause the heart to fail. However, high blood pressure is also a consequence of high resistance in the circulation – that is, arteries become clogged and inflexible, so the heart has to work harder and is under greater strain in its task of pumping blood round the body. The clogging of arteries (commonly called atherosclerosis) is made worse by there being too much fat in the diet, being overweight or smoking – all of which are physical stresses. However, there is evidence that it can also be made worse by stresses created by the personality of the sufferer. Those who are ambitious, driven, competitive, impatient, hostile and work under great time pressure, were summarized as being Type A personalities by Rosenman and Friedman (1961) and it is people in this group who are most likely to have coronary heart disease. However, there is much more to personality than the Type A label – and its lazy, laid-back opposite, Type B – and this is discussed in the next chapter.

Cancer has sometimes been linked to stress, but clear evidence of a relationship does not exist. In cancer, cells in the body do not die but grow without any control until they destroy other cells. Although stress can lead to the death of cells, we have no direct evidence that it stimulates their uncontrolled growth. The causes of only a few types of cancer are known and we cannot put the rest down to stress. Nevertheless, there are some dramatic instances in which inoperable cancer has apparently been cured without any explanation and there is now an abundance of evidence that shows that mental attitude to cancer can have a major effect on its course. Those who give up have a much worse outcome than those who fight, and stress has a part to play in this.

Stress pretending to be disease

Stress can also cause symptoms that fool us into thinking we have physical disease when we are really quite well. Our sympathetic nervous systems stimulate our bodies and produce feelings that are very similar to those of real disease. The irritating awareness of the heart beating (and missing beats), difficulty in breathing, nausea and sickness, tension in arms and legs, headache and giddiness, interfere with our thoughts and actions. We often feel anxious and upset at these times. It annoys us because there is often no reason to feel anxious. Sometimes only one or two of these bodily feelings bother us and most of our anxiety is about these symptoms. When this happens, it is very easy to get the idea that there is an undetected physical illness causing these symptoms. The body is behaving in an unfamiliar way that is alarming, so an appointment is made with the doctor to have a full physical check-up. (It is interesting that people with other health problems seldom ask for this; they just present their symptoms.) Now this may seem a perfectly reasonable thing to do, but, in most cases, the outcome of the consultation is far from satisfactory. The doctor examines you, finds no evidence of physical illness and reassures you that all is well. At one level you are pleased, but, at another, you are suspicious. If you have no physical disease, then what is the cause of these nasty feelings? You blurt out the question, 'You don't think I'm imagining this, do you, doctor?' You don't want to appear to be wasting the doctor's time and yet you want more than simple reassurance. You may even feel angry or suspect the doctor of incompetence.

In fact, your doctor is in a difficult position. There is no way to be absolutely sure that you have no physical disease but, from the pattern of your symptoms, it is much more likely that they have been caused by stress. This does not mean that the symptoms are imaginary. They are real to you and there are genuine changes in the body, but they are not the changes that occur as a result of a physical disease, at least not at this stage. If your doctor is not sure about this, and particularly if you go back repeatedly with the same complaint, you may be referred to a specialist at a hospital. The specialist has the advantages of a fuller range of tests and expert knowledge. So if, for example, you have palpitations, you are likely to be referred to a heart specialist. The specialist carries out all the tests necessary to make sure you have no heart disease and again reassures you. Often, strangely, this reassurance is no more satisfying than the reassurance you got from your own doctor, unless of course by this time your symptoms have gone away. The danger is that you will start on a round of medical (and non-medical) consultations, hoping that one of them will find your undiscovered disease. If you persevere long enough (and spend enough money), you may finally have the 'disease' named. However, it is not a real disease and the name may just be a description of your main problem in Latin and Greek – a name that sounds impressive but says very little.

If your doctor recognizes that these feelings are related to psychological stresses, there may still be some difficulty in talking about them to you. The mere mention of the word 'psychological' implies to some people that they are imagining their symptoms and they are 'neurotic'. So, however the interview goes, it is likely that you will be far from satisfied with your visit. If you become upset and angry, your symptoms will trouble you still more and so you may feel worse after the interview than you did before.

Doctors used to call these complaints 'psychosomatic' or 'functional' disorders, but they are now given the rather unsatisfactory name of 'somatoform disorders' – that is, the mental distress is converted into a somatic (bodily) form and this fools the sufferer into thinking there is a coexisting physical disease. Among these is the condition 'hypochondriasis', now sometimes renamed 'health anxiety' – worry about having a disease even when the doctor can find no evidence of one. This is now recognized as a big part of medical practice, with about 1 in 12 of all people seeing doctors having health anxiety rather than real disease. It is one of the problems now being treated by the therapies discussed later in the book (Hawton, Salkovskis, et al., 1989).

Do these symptoms that masquerade as disease, but are really mental distress, cause real disease if they go on for long enough? This is a question that naturally follows from what we have said earlier about stress, but, curiously, the answer seems to be no. People can go on for years worrying about their hearts skipping beats, pumping like steam hammers and making the chest feel sore without real heart disease developing, and the same applies to other symptoms. Some doctors feel that it might even be of value to have these symptoms because they warn you when you are doing too much and make sure you pace yourself in all your activities. So, although it may seem strange, the people who are often most worried about their bodies are the ones who should have the least cause for concern. Having said that, we cannot regard these feelings as healthy – they cause worry and annoyance and we would love to be rid of them. However, most of the ill health affects the mind rather than the organs in the body. I am not just putting out the doctor's usual line of reassurance here: there is no connection between the bodily feelings of stress we have been looking at and physical disease.

Stress can be involved in the cause of physical disease and the first evidence of disease is a bodily symptom. It may be the pain of a duodenal ulcer, the headache and sickness of migraine or the difficulty in breathing of the asthmatic. Emotional stress alone does not cause any of these diseases; they are due to a combination of factors. However, emotional stress alone is the most frequent cause of psychosomatic complaints.

Once a disease has developed, emotional factors can make it worse and the diseases that are commonest are those affecting the parts of the body most closely involved with the stimulation of the sympathetic nervous system. So it is advisable for people with heart disease to avoid all types of emotional stress whenever they can because it makes extra demands on the heart, but no such advice needs to be given in anaemia as it is not affected by the emotions. Asthma, bowel and skin disease, high blood pressure, peptic ulcer and migraine are all sensitive to emotional pressures and relapses can be caused by them. It is much easier to make changes to the diet, take tablets or move to a new part of the country than it is to cut down on stress, but it can be done.

Stress in response to events

Stress is often felt most keenly in the mind rather than the body and when we are faced with tragedy or other dramatic changes in our lives we can usually recognize the source of the stress quite clearly.

However, there are many ways in which stress can show itself. It is particularly difficult to adjust to severe changes if they catch us unprepared. If a close relative dies suddenly, we are faced with immediate and severe stress. We are forced to adjust to a change that has happened unexpectedly. Such adjustment is painful and hard, but usually we adapt in the end. Sometimes, though, if the task seems too much, we take the easy way out. Although at one level we accept the loss, at an emotional level we pretend it has not happened. The distress and unhappiness that we should be feeling is not shown at all. People note how well we are taking the loss because we do not give an embarrassing public display of emotion and the stiff upper lip appears to have won again. Whether it has or not is debatable. Is it best to suppress the distressing emotions rumbling like a volcano ready to erupt or is it preferable to let them be expressed? The answer is, as for so many difficult problems in life, neither one nor the other, but both to some degree. The extremes of both approaches are illustrated by the conditions of shell shock and post-traumatic stress disorder.

Shell shock

'Shell shock' is a term that was developed during World War I. It was used to describe the phenomenon observed in soldiers who developed severe mental breakdowns in the trenches of Belgium and France when they were constantly bombarded with shell-fire from enemy lines. What life under such conditions must have been like is very hard for most of us to conceive in our more pampered times. Then, soldiers lived for months in intolerable conditions under constant threat of death. The terrible cry 'over the top', when they had to advance out of the safety of the trenches and run towards the enemy, meant death for many and those who lived only exchanged one set of squalid conditions for another.

A shell arriving out of the sky and exploding close to you, killing and wounding almost at random, is a remarkably stressful experience. Small wonder, then, that the natural protective reaction was to go backwards rather than forwards, 'back down the line' rather than over the top. Duty and instinct were in conflict and, at times, instinct won. So, the affected soldier went into a state in which he forgot who and where he was or what he was doing and walked instinctively backwards from the trenches in a daze, a state that we now describe as 'dissociation' – the splitting off of part of our mind (or body) from the rest, so that duty and instinct could be kept in separate compartments.

Unfortunately, the subtlety of this distinction was not noticed by the military authorities and, indeed, not by the medical ones either at the beginning of the war. So many of the poor sufferers, far from getting help to come to terms with their intolerable stress, received a different form of management – they were executed for desertion. So much, therefore, for the stiff upper lip approach to mental distress and the policy of totally useless killings that only justifies Voltaire's mocking phrase describing the purpose of similar executions 100 years earlier, 'pour encourager les autres' – 'to encourage the others'. The contrast today could not be greater. Counsellors would come from every corner, offering help and support after people had experienced stress of this magnitude.

Post-traumatic stress disorder

In the last edition of this book, the term 'post-traumatic stress disorder', now often abbreviated to PTSD, was never mentioned. Now it is on everybody's lips as its prominence in the media makes ignorance of it almost impossible. What has happened in the last 20 years?

The simple answer is Vietnam, and American guilt. Before the Vietnam War, soldiers had fought bravely in battles since the time organized combat began; ordinary people had coped with the natural disasters of earthquakes, typhoons and tidal waves, floods and hurricanes; nurses and doctors had fought to save lives at times of epidemics, such as the plague in Europe and the influenza pandemic of 1918; and victims of torture, abuse and harsh imprisonment had suffered long before Alexander Solzhenitsyn graphically represented the sufferings of those imprisoned in the Russian Gulag.

So why was Vietnam different? The answer is a combination of American angst at being on a losing side in a war for the first time in its short history, a resurgent American psychiatric movement that got a buzz out of new diagnoses, encapsulated in the publication of the third edition of the *Diagnostic and Statistical Manual of Mental Disorders* (DSM-III) in 1980 by the American Psychiatric Association, and what Ben Shephard, a journalist who has made an impressive study of the history of military stress, describes as 'an American public guilty at having sent veterans to a dirty, unwinnable war' (Shephard, 2002).

These three elements might seem to have little natural connection, but they actually linked together at this time very closely. If you look at the problems of the returning Vietnam veterans and the desperate search for a solution for them, you can see how the three issues of defeat, labelling and guilt become linked. Soldiers from Vietnam did not return as conquering heroes; they had lost a war. Neither were they piped back as noble in defeat as those who were in the British Army and evacuated from Dunkirk in 1940. They were an embarrassment and nobody wanted to know them. The words 'army veteran' until then had always been a source of pride, even though they rested somewhat uneasily on young men who were not yet 30. Even my great-great-uncle, Samuel, who played his part in the American Civil War during the Battle of the Wilderness in Virginia in 1865, was proud to be considered a veteran, despite being of Irish blood.

However, a society that felt both guilty and uncomfortable about those it had sent into battle could not ignore them when they returned. It was even more disturbing that so many had major problems in adjusting to life away from the scene of battle. So, up on a white charger, rode the American Psychiatric Association with its new diagnosis – post-traumatic stress disorder. By so doing, it introduced the new science – some call it an industry – of 'traumatology'. This is the special knowledge of not physical wounds, but ones to the psyche, appropriately first described by the American philosopher and psychologist William James in 1890 in his *The Principles of Psychology*.

This new diagnosis, PTSD (it is now better known in abbreviation than in full), described a set of characteristic symptoms that followed extreme mental trauma, defined as 'an event that is outside the range of usual human experience and that would be markedly distressing to almost anyone' (American Psychiatric Association, 1980). The symptoms included 'recurrent and intrusive distressing recollections of the event', such as distressing dreams, the sudden feeling 'as if the traumatic event were recurring', such as episodes of flashbacks, and 'intense distress at exposure to events that symbolize or represent the traumatic event' in whole or in part.

You can now see why this new diagnosis was a godsend. At a stroke it could explain why the Vietnam veterans were having such difficulties after they returned home and could also assuage the guilt of a population that had sent them away in the first place. These people were ill and needed therapy. Post-traumatic stress disorder was the new form of shell shock and, now that it had been properly diagnosed, it could be treated in the same way as other illnesses. It could be treated with special forms of psychological therapy specifically tailored to the condition, the most popular of which was debriefing.

'Debriefing' – a systematic form of counselling after severe, traumatic events – seemed to be the therapeutic strategy linked to post-traumatic stress. The notion was that, by exploring the events linked to the trauma in a quiet and non-judgemental way, grief and other emotions could be expressed safely, leading to resolution of the problem and prevention of recurrence. This was such an obvious solution that it seemed unethical not to give it whenever there was a major tragedy. So, whenever there was such a tragedy, grief and trauma counsellors were quickly on the scene to pick up the pieces and provide the care that was so sorely needed.

Unfortunately, this new commonsense treatment is no more appropriate than executing people with shell shock. The results are, at best, no different from doing nothing apart from giving simple reassurance and, more commonly, people after major trauma are usually made worse by debriefing, particularly in the longer term (Mayou, et al., 2000).

The tragedy of PTSD is that it medicalizes a problem that is primarily concerned with adjustment. Indeed, the condition is one of the adjustment disorders in the mental health classification and one of the best ways of promoting successful adjustment is to take responsibility for your own destiny and not hand it over to apparent experts who are largely whistling in the dark.

I will take one example – my own profession. I am a community psychiatrist working in inner London. This involves visiting people at all hours. I am abused several times daily, my parentage questioned repeatedly, am frequently spat on and physically attacked occasionally, but this goes with the territory. My colleagues are put under similar pressures and we do what we can to learn ways of avoiding or escaping from such conflict without injury. Yet, when I read of soldiers suing the Army because of their experiences of death, paramedics claiming compensation for their experiences with accident victims and teachers retiring early and claiming extra payments because of aggressive behaviour by their pupils, I am sad. Although the obvious question 'What did they expect?' can naturally be asked, it is the knowledge that only the complete phoneys who have simulated their symptoms will ever benefit even if they win their cases that is hard to bear. The remainder will suffer more because they have both handed over responsibility to someone else for their problems and are going down the road of blaming and claiming, so they will be reinforcing their own suffering and reminding themselves of an unpleasant past rather than working towards a positive future.

The saddest action of all is when those who suffer trauma sue whatever organization they deem to be responsible for 'not providing proper counselling' at the time. As such counselling is ineffective or even counter-productive, it might be more appropriate to sue for the damaging effects of counselling (although if this is given in good faith and with consent such action would hardly be justified). So, please keep PTSD in proportion and try to avoid using the term unless you are involved with the legal side of PTSD, in which case the financial benefit that is almost sure to follow has to be balanced against the knowledge that your action may be doing harm.

Stress and anxiety

Stress and anxiety are closely related but are not the same. Anxiety is almost always in either the foreground or background of any stress problem, but it should be seen more as a fuel for stress rather than its equivalent. Just as cutting off the supply of fuel will stop a car or any machinery that is out of control, cutting down and controlling levels of anxiety will usually be beneficial for stress.

Although fear and anxiety are usually very easy to detect, they can play tricks from time to time. Many people do not remember everything about a serious accident, fire or similar episode, even though they were conscious all the time. The sight of bodies being crushed or burnt and the cries of agony and distress are too much for our senses to bear. So, at the time, we shut them off from consciousness. Oddly enough, if we actually do lose consciousness, symptoms such as PTSD are less likely than if we stayed conscious the whole time.

Occasionally, we do the wrong things by not responding to the messages from our senses. When people are said to be paralysed with fear they are often not frightened at all on the surface, but so overwhelmed by anxiety that they do nothing. Like a computer or electrical instrument that is overloaded, they suspend normal activity and wait. This can have disastrous consequences.

It has been suspected that lives are lost unnecessarily when aeroplanes crash-land and catch fire. Even when there is time for all the passengers to escape through the emergency chutes, some stay glued to their seats with the safety belts securely fixed. They cannot adjust quickly enough to the change from being relaxed and secure to an emergency in which their lives can be saved only by their own reactions. The transfer of complete faith in the air crew back to personal responsibility for one's own safety takes place too quickly and, while they may respond to instructions from others, they are incapable of thinking for themselves. It is only helpful to be calm in the face of danger if we fully realize what the danger is and how we are going to deal with it.

Anxiety is not always harmful. Short-term feelings of anxiety are often helpful, even though they may seem unpleasant at the time. Students working for an exam are likely to work harder if they are anxious about doing well than if they are not bothered about it. The journalist who is made anxious because she has to write a story in time for the next edition of the paper is likely to work most efficiently when the deadline is approaching. The father who is anxious about his daughter playing in the road will move her to a safer place and so reduce the risk of an accident. The list is endless, and without anxiety all our lives would be the poorer.

In harmful stress, anxiety can become so crippling that it stops us from doing anything constructive. Students who have an abnormal fear of examinations (a phobia) become so anxious about tests that they go to pieces. They look at the question paper and find the words have no meaning. They cannot remember all the work that they have spent many weeks revising. When they raise their pen to write, their hand shakes so much every word is illegible. A little anxiety is good for us but too much is deadly. Once it gets out of hand, it seems to be with us constantly. Instead of being turned on by demand, it surrounds us like a cloud. When this happens, we cannot say what we are anxious about and make feeble excuses to satisfy others. However, in reality, every little change is taken as a serious threat. The sudden noise of a bell ringing, a knock on the door, an innocent item on the television, a telephone call, are all full of hidden dangers and create still more anxiety. It is as though we are stumbling through a dark tunnel, not knowing where we are going and what horrors lie ahead, so every signal, no matter how small, fills us with foreboding.

The most severe form of anxiety is panic. Recently this has been given the diagnostic label 'panic disorder'. This is, in my view, a mistake, as panic is part of the anxious spectrum, not something separate from it. We all have the capacity for panic – the feeling of dread of approaching catastrophe accompanied by shaking, sweating, palpitations and the urgent wish to escape from something we know not what. However, panic is not a disease, it is often a reaction to something that has happened to us that we do not recognize fully. Recently I saw someone who had their first attack of panic at the age of 79. It came out of the blue and terrified and troubled her to such an extent that she felt death would be preferable to the possibility of further attacks. However, when it became clear that there was a cause (an undiscovered chest infection that responded well to antibiotics, but had lowered both her physical and psychological defences), she was able to bring it under control and realize it was not a separate disease.

If anxiety persists for very long, we become inefficient shadows of our normal selves. First, the anxiety extends into the night and this shows itself as insomnia. We cannot get to sleep until the anxieties of the day have subsided, which can take many hours if we have been strung up by them all day. The consequent lack of sleep leads to poor concentration and efficiency the next day and this makes us even more anxious. We also become irritable and often quite different from our normal personalities. We snap and snarl, find fault with everyone except ourselves and get involved in petty arguments that waste even more time. Although we get angry with ourselves for behaving in this kind of way, we do not seem to be able to prevent it. Because we are not coping, we can easily get downhearted and depressed. We feel sorry for ourselves, feel like crying, think the future seems hopeless and lose all energy. This

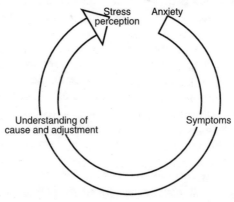

The virtuous circle of stress feedback

24

makes us cope even less well than before. So, instead of adjusting to the change, we make it worse by giving the wrong sort of feedback.

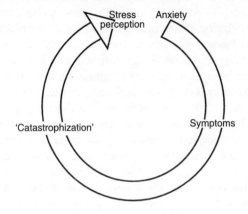

The vicious circle of stress feedback

'Feedback' is essentially an engineering term and we need to be quite clear what it means. When something changes in a system, feedback can make the change less intrusive (often called a servo mechanism in engineering as it stabilizes by compensating for the change) or more intrusive (which aggravates the problem and leads to a lack of equilibrium). Most healthy stress involves feedback leading to adjustment and only lasts a short time, constituting the virtuous circle of stress feedback. In effect, the stress leads to symptoms that serve as a warning; the warning is heeded and corrective action is taken so there is little perception of stress. My panic patient moved rapidly into this virtuous circle once it became clear that her chest infection was the real cause of her panic, not some obscure biochemical predisposition.

The opposite, vicious circle of stress feedback replaces the virtuous one when the symptoms are not properly understood and interpreted as something terrible. This is sometimes given the complex word 'catastrophization' – the ultimate mountain made from the smallest of molehills. Each element of stress reinforces the next in line so the perception of stress goes on building until it becomes enormous.

To use another metaphor, the problem is like a snowball rolling down a hill. To begin with it is small and manageable, but, as it rolls, it grows larger, picking up more and more snow, and, as it becomes heavier, it gets out of control and thunders on to destruction. It is this process that leads to the change we commonly call a nervous breakdown. This is not a formal medical term, but it aptly describes the state we get into. The normal mechanisms of our mental function become overloaded and then stop working. Even though the breakdown may seem to have no purpose, it at least stops us from doing more damage to ourselves and is often the signpost to recovery. However, because it happens at a time when everything is out of control, it leads to actions that may be completely out of character. Many people seem to realize at one level of their minds that something must be done to stop themselves rushing headlong from crisis to crisis and bring the final act of breakdown on themselves.

The upright housewife who has always been the best of citizens takes goods from a shop without paying for them, the quiet respectable worker who normally caves in to authority gives his employer a punch in the ribs, the proper young lady who is a stickler for etiquette takes an overdose of pills and finishes up with the indignity of the stomach pump. It seems as though the only way we can put a stop to such self-generating stress is by doing something that is quite the opposite of our normal behaviour. And it works. Although the immediate consequences of a breakdown are unpleasant, they allow us to look at our problem in a different light, see things that we were blind to before, realize that blaming outside influences for our troubles was wrong, that we alone were responsible. Crises have a habit of clearing away the cobwebs so we can see things more clearly and get them into perspective.

Most of the harmful stress we come across in life is of this type. We ask too much of ourselves when we are under pressure. Our bodies and minds cannot keep up with the speed and intensity of the demands we make on them. It would be wrong, however, to assume that stress only results from too much pressure. Equally severe stress can result from too little stimulation. Some may find this hard to believe, but it is only because there are relatively few people who have been severely understimulated. When people have been placed in situations of this kind, commonly described as sensory deprivation (Zubek, 1969), they react in a most surprising way.

Imagine being suspended in a tank of warm water with your head covered and a breathing mask over your face, with sound-proofing to remove all noise and your eyes blindfolded. This may sound a blissful way of whiling away the hours, but it turns out not to be. Very few people can tolerate these conditions for more than a few hours because the feelings they experience are so unpleasant. In the absence of stimulation, our nervous systems create mischief. There is great difficulty in concentrating, our minds wander and odd ideas and fantasies confuse our thinking. Often these are sexual ones, as one might imagine when suspended in water, but although these might appear to be pleasant (particularly to younger men whose appetite for sexual fantasy is ravenous), they quickly become distorted and unpleasant.

Time gets out of joint, so minutes seem like hours, sleep and waking come and go and there may be intolerable boredom. Prolonged understimulation of the senses leads to hallucinations, particularly visual ones of bright cartoon-like objects that are sinister – more like pink porcupines than white rabbits – and can also be very frightening. More than a third of the volunteers for these experiments, most of which took place in the 1960s, found the experiences so intolerable that they left the experiments early. Often they were amazed to find that they had only been confined for a few hours. Instead of feeling continuously relaxed, a proportion of subjects felt tense, with headaches and other pains. Some even developed symptoms of frank psychosis, feeling that the shape of their bodies was changing and believing that their thoughts were being controlled by other people.

So, when these people come back to normal life again, they often talk about their experiences as though they had been through the severe stress of armed battle. Although this may at first seem odd, when we consider our definition of stress, it is entirely predictable. Stress, you will remember, is the reaction of the mind and body to change, and change can be up or down, less or more. Even the proverbial man who goes on banging his head against a brick wall experiences a minor form of stress when he stops using his head as a hammer, although it is much less than if he continues. Most change that results in less stimulation than previously is mildly pleasurable, but if the difference is great and if understimulation is prolonged, the mind and body react in just the same stressful way as when they are overstimulated. Although it is not every day that you are likely to have the opportunity of being suspended in warm water with only a breathing tube for company or even lying in a sound-proofed room, you will probably have experienced situations in real life that are similar if not so extreme. Boredom is often the first sign of

27

understimulation, and who can claim that he or she has never been bored? If you are bored and relaxed, you can escape further boredom by dropping off to sleep, but if you already have had more than enough sleep it is another matter. Often when convalescing from an illness we go through a stage when we feel fit but are still confined to bed. We are fed up with reading, writing letters or doing crosswords and we can think of nothing that we would like more than to stretch our legs and take a walk in the open air. This is the stage of illness we often find most frustrating, and during which we are the most difficult of patients. We are irritable and snappy, complain of tension, aches and pains, and show all the signs of harmful stress.

The same stressful effects are shown whenever we are forced to go on doing the same thing for week after week without any prospect of change. This is the curious paradox of stress. Although it is the reaction to change, it can also be the reaction to lack of change. This is because a life that repeats itself in the same predictable way as the hands of a clock retracing each minute and hour of the day becomes a life of boredom and understimulation. Every movement and act is predictable and eventually becomes automatic, and the parts of you that want change become increasingly frustrated. A life of necessary novelty becomes one of breathtaking boredom and the harmful stress cycle is set in motion.

Unfortunately, far too many of us think that we are compelled to go through life without much change. We do things that we would prefer not to do and, after a little while, cannot see any alternative. There are ways of escaping the deadlock of boredom and these are discussed later. At this stage we need to be reminded that, although the highly pressured business executive tends to come to mind whenever we think of stress, exactly the same degree of stress can be experienced by a bored housewife, spending her day cleaning, shopping and preparing meals in a continuous round of duty, with very little time spent on her own needs. If she would choose to do none of these things if she had alternatives and if her family take her for granted so that she never gets any respite, she and her executive equivalent will both be paying visits to the doctor because they are experiencing the effects of stress, be these physical or mental.

Each of us has a level of stress with which we are most happy, one that satisfies our need for novelty yet allows us to make adjustments to change smoothly and completely. Because we differ from each other, we should not allow others to decide this level for us. We are not prepackaged machines set to operate at the flick of a switch, although the speeches of politicians, the slogans of advertising and the techniques of mass communication sometimes assume we are. The pressures on us to conform have always been great in human society, but now it is not so much the heavy hand of the dictator as soft talking through the television screen and 'keeping up with the Joneses' that is the main threat to our independence. If we give in to these pressures, about half of us will find that the stresses we come across are at, or near to, our optimum level, but the other half will find they are either too low or too high. To decide whether or not the stress in your life is healthy or harmful, there is no alternative to using yourself as the yardstick. By all means listen to what others have to say, but remember that you are the only one who feels your symptoms of stress and so you are in the best position to judge if they are doing harm.

So, how do you decide on the ideal level of stress for you? In this book it is argued that personality is the key. 'Personality' is not a showbiz term that pretends to tell you whether or not you have star quality, but a word describing the sort of person you are, the ultimate you, stripped of pretence and humbug. Now you may have very clear ideas about the sort of person you are. Alternatively, you may think of personality as a meaningless term thought up by psychologists. Whatever your views, read the next chapter with an open mind and prepare to learn something more about yourself.

3

Stress and personality

When we are asked to describe someone's personality, we often find
it difficult. The questioner is asking what kind of person is X or Y
and while it is easy to describe their physical appearance, it is
difficult to put personality into words. We often finish up using
bland words such as nice, pleasant, all right and OK, which mean
virtually nothing. Yet, we all have a mental image of someone's
personality, the particular combination of features that is as unique
as a fingerprint and much more interesting. While everyone is
different, there are some features that tend to go together and form
types of personality.

If you would like to find out your type of personality, you should
answer the questionnaire that follows. For each item you are given
seven possible replies (indicated by the letters a to g). Decide which
of the seven comes closest to describing your reaction and note this
as your *first* choice. If you wish, you can also do the same again after
deciding your *second* and *third* choices. Try to take your past
experience as well as your present feelings into account before
making your answer. Please answer as honestly as possible – there
are no right or wrong replies. Even if none of the replies fits your
particular reaction, pick the one (or three if you decide to do so) that
are closest.

Personality questionnaire

1 You are in a hurry and about to cross a busy road in a large town.
   Do you:

   (a) feel angry with drivers if you are kept waiting?
   (b) only cross when the way is quite clear, no matter how long
       you have to wait?
   (c) only cross when other people are crossing?
   (d) rush across, dodging the traffic?
   (e) only cross when traffic has stopped moving as drivers can
       never be trusted?
   (f) try to get the traffic to stop, making it clear that you are in a
       hurry?

(g) look for a zebra crossing (or similar special crossing for pedestrians) and cross there even if it means a detour?

2 You are offered alcoholic drinks at a party where most of the guests are strangers to you. Do you:

(a) accept one drink but rarely accept a second?
(b) accept the drink that most of the others are drinking?
(c) drink until you feel calm and more confident?
(d) drink as much as you can get?
(e) refuse the drink unless you know exactly what is in it?
(f) drink until you feel happy?
(g) refuse the offer?

3 You have a choice of jobs, each with similar pay. Which of the following would you consider important in making your choice:

(a) good prospects of promotion?
(b) easy work that makes few demands on you?
(c) security?
(d) good holidays?
(e) working alone?
(f) working with people who understand you?
(g) a set routine?

4 You are waiting in a queue and there is no immediate prospect of the queue moving. Do you:

(a) keep looking at your watch and become impatient?
(b) just relax while waiting?
(c) worry about one thing or another?
(d) prefer not to wait and do something else instead?
(e) look at other people in the queue?
(f) talk to other people in the queue?
(g) work out problems in your mind while waiting?

5 You have just been told that you have won first prize in a lottery. Is your immediate reaction to:

(a) work out how you will spend your winnings?
(b) continue what you were doing as though nothing had happened?
(c) take something to calm you down?
(d) have a party to celebrate?
(e) worry about possible publicity?

(f) tell a close friend or relative?
(g) check the number of the lottery ticket?

6 You have just been interviewed for a new job and told you were unsuccessful. Do you:

(a) feel angry because they did not appreciate your true worth?
(b) forget about it immediately?
(c) feel tense and miserable?
(d) go and have a drink to forget about it?
(e) feel the interviewer had a grudge against you?
(f) get it off your chest by talking to somebody about it?
(g) go over the interview in your mind to see where you went wrong?

7 You have just had an argument with a friend and are not on speaking terms. Do you:

(a) forget about it by concentrating hard on something else?
(b) take it in your stride and ignore it?
(c) find it difficult to stop yourself shaking?
(d) feel like hitting somebody?
(e) wonder why people seem to turn against you?
(f) tell someone else what happened?
(g) go over the argument again and again in your mind?

8 You are planning a holiday. Do you:

(a) go somewhere new that presents a challenge?
(b) go where you can rest and relax?
(c) go somewhere that is safe and secure?
(d) make no plans and hope for the best?
(e) prefer to go where you can be on your own?
(f) decide where you are going, but leave the details to someone else?
(g) prefer to plan in detail so that every day is accounted for?

9 A close member of your family has failed to arrive home at the expected time. Do you:

(a) use the opportunity to catch up on some work?
(b) feel unconcerned?
(c) get very worried indeed?
(d) only realize that he or she is late after they arrive home?
(e) feel suspicious about the reasons for the delay?
(f) feel all right as long as there is someone else to talk to?

(g) work out in your mind all the possible causes for the delay?

10 You are about to buy some new clothes. Do you choose:

(a) the best clothes, even if they are the most expensive?
(b) clothes that are the most comfortable?
(c) clothes that are in your nearest shop, even if they are not ideal?
(d) the first clothes that take your fancy?
(e) clothes that are such that you do not stand out in a crowd?
(f) the latest fashion?
(g) clothes that are very similar to your present ones?

11 You have just been informed that a close friend of yours has been injured in an accident. Is your reaction to:

(a) get details of the accident and organize help?
(b) reassure others as much as possible?
(c) feel very upset?
(d) feel glad that it was not you?
(e) find out who was to blame?
(f) visit him or her as soon as possible?
(g) work out in your mind how it could have been avoided?

12 You have just been introduced to a stranger you will be working with closely in the future. Would you like them to be someone:

(a) with ambition, energy and drive?
(b) who is easy-going and placid?
(c) who makes you feel at ease?
(d) who is lively and exciting?
(e) you can trust?
(f) who is interesting to talk to?
(g) who is reliable and conscientious?

13 You are working and have just been presented with an unusual problem. Do you:

(a) have to get it sorted out before you can return to your normal work?
(b) deal with it in exactly the same way as your ordinary work?
(c) find it upsets your concentration?
(d) prefer dealing with it instead of doing your ordinary work?
(e) make certain it is your responsibility before dealing with it?
(f) usually ask advice before dealing with it?
(g) only deal with it when you have completely finished the work you are doing?

14 You have nearly finished work for the day and have a severe headache. Do you:

  (a) take a painkiller and keep on working until the job is done no matter how bad your headache is?
  (b) stop working and rest until the headache goes away?
  (c) take a painkiller and something to calm your nerves?
  (d) have an alcoholic drink?
  (e) think you have been made to work too hard?
  (f) take a painkiller immediately and lie down until it takes effect?
  (g) stop work temporarily, but continue as soon as the headache is better?

15 You are listening to somebody who takes a long time to explain things. Do you:

  (a) try to work out what he means and interrupt him by repeating your interpretation so that you save time?
  (b) wait until he has finished no matter how long he or she takes?
  (c) worry when you will be allowed to speak?
  (d) interrupt and talk about something completely different?
  (e) wonder if he or she is making fun of you?
  (f) stop listening, but pretend to be still listening?
  (g) listen carefully to everything that is said and reorganize it in your mind?

Scoring

Now add up the total scores for each separate letter throughout the questionnaire. If you have made one choice, only just give one for each of the scores. If you have chosen three answers for each of the questions, then for each first choice score three points, for each second choice, two points and for each third choice, one point. The letter with the highest number of points indicates your personality type. The types and their matching letters are:

  (a) ambitious type   (e) suspicious type
  (b) placid type   (f) dependent type
  (c) worrying type   (g) fussy type.
  (d) carefree type

The advantage of the second method is that, if you get equal scores for two personality types, you can add up the total of first choices for

34

each of them and choose the one that has the most. Using the first method, you have to choose which type of personality seems to fit you best.

All these personality types have unattractive as well as pleasant features, but I would like you to stay with the type that the questionnaire has decided for you, even if you feel it is not an accurate one. You can make a decision at the end as to whether or not it is really correct after all.

Let us take a closer look at each of these personalities. I am going to describe some typical examples of each one – the kinds of people who would score 10 or more points (using the single choice method) or 30 or more points (using the three choices method) for the personality indicated in the questionnaire. To match with the letters from the questionnaire, each one is named after the first seven letters of the Greek alphabet (the sex allocation is at random).

Personality types

The ambitious type

Ms Alpha has done well in life. She has always been active and energetic. She cannot stand to be still for more than a few minutes and, when she is not working, she is always busy with one activity or another. She is conscientious and has very high standards, so often is annoyed with others for not coming up to her expectations. Time is a problem in her life – she never seems to have enough. At work, she is always rushing from one appointment to another and has no time to relax. She becomes impatient easily, talks quickly and aggressively and tends to frighten people. She is dominant in her relationships and likes to control those around her. Because she has worked so hard and had so much energy, she is now the managing director of her company, which has become a much larger concern since she took over. People are proud of what she has done, but wish she would take things a little easier now.

The placid type

Mr Beta is a quiet man – many people say he is lazy. Although he did well at school, he did not like the idea of further education with more examinations and took a job as a farm labourer. He is now a market gardener and has a reasonable standard of living, but his wife keeps telling him how much better off they would be if only he worked harder. Often in the summer, when he should be busy in the garden, he says the weather is too good for work and goes off to the seaside with his family. His favourite hobby is fishing and he spends hours at a canal near his home, even though he never catches anything of importance. He is bad with money and his wife has to keep the accounts or bills are not paid. He never seems to worry about anything and is seldom involved in arguments. Because of these traits some people find him boring. Although he has always been good at sport, he has never won any competitions and cannot see the point of them. He says he does things because he enjoys doing them and for no other reason.

The worrying type

Miss Gamma has always been 'highly strung'. She has little self-confidence and from an early age has been worried about doing things wrong. Even when everything is going well, she is worried about the future and consequently finds it difficult to relax. She likes to organize her life so that she can avoid being faced with new problems, which only make her nervous. However, as life is unpredictable and she is not a very good organizer, she usually finds that whenever there is a crisis or unexpected hitch in her life, she becomes very panicky and sometimes feels as if she will go to pieces. She works as a secretary and, although she has been told she is a good one, she cannot really believe it and is always worried that she might be about to let people down.

She used to think that she would feel more confident once she was in control of her job, but it never seemed to happen. Although she is capable of getting a better post, she is worried about the strain of increased responsibility and prefers to stay in her present position. She has been engaged to be married for a year. Her boyfriend is very understanding, but, at times, they have had serious disagreements – chiefly about sex. She is afraid that she might be frigid and has avoided sexual relations because of her doubts and fears, although she pretends to her boyfriend that her decision is a moral one. At times she wonders if she can cope with marriage and also doubts her ability to look after children. Whenever she looks into the future, troubles seem to be crowding in on her.

The carefree type

Mr Delta is a DJ at a local radio station, but he has also worked as a van driver, racing mechanic and salesman. His favourite saying is 'variety is the spice of life' and he acts on this by moving around the country from one job to another. His friends keep advising him to think about the future and settle down, but he cannot understand their concern. He enjoys life now and does not see why the future should be any different. In his spare time, he likes parachute jumping and hang-gliding and especially relishes the feeling of flying apparently unsupported through the air. He had hoped to go into rally driving when he was a mechanic, but had so many driving accidents that no insurance company would cover him. He liked the excitement and novelty of his job as a DJ at first, but now he is beginning to find this a little tedious and already is thinking of another change. He drinks more alcohol than most people and is sometimes violent when he has had too much. He has had many girlfriends in the past, but usually ended each relationship after a few months. Two of his girlfriends became pregnant and claimed that he was the father, but he denied this absolutely (he is worried that they might ask for a DNA test, though). He tells all his girlfriends that he has no intention of getting married, but they still become closely involved with him. The thought of living with one person for the rest of his life makes him shudder.

The suspicious type

Mr Epsilon is a schoolteacher. He is dedicated to his job and takes it very seriously. He actually feels more at home with children than he does with adults. Since his early years, he has been concerned about what people think of him and cannot help thinking that they criticize him behind his back. He distrusts most people and is careful not to reveal his true feelings until he knows someone really well. When he is criticized, he takes it very badly and thinks about it for weeks afterwards. Even when he is not being criticized, he finds double meanings in things that are said to him and always takes the least favourable interpretation. His wife has to be careful what she says to him because he bears a grudge easily and, if annoyed, he often refuses to talk to her for days on end. Whenever he has moved house or changed to a new school, it has taken many months for him to settle down and he goes through a phase when he is even more prickly and sensitive than usual. If he is asked to take on different duties at school, he thinks that he is being criticized for being incompetent and becomes moody. However, at home with his family he is usually settled and relaxed, and is happiest when playing with his children. He trusts his wife most of the time, but, when he is in his more suspicious moods, he gets very jealous. Although he trusts her in one sense, he often wonders what she is doing during the day and makes frequent telephone calls to confirm where she is. Despite his suspicious nature, once he makes friends, they remain friends for life and he will do anything for them.

The dependent type

Miss Zeta is a fashion model. She wanted to be a ballet dancer when she was young, but the strain of constant practice and physical exercise was too much for her and she drifted into modelling. She is glad she made the move and only regrets that her career cannot be a long one. At present, she knows that she is attractive and gets a great deal of attention from male admirers, but fears that nobody really knows, least of all herself, what she is really like. She has always liked being the centre of interest and her job satisfies these needs. She is also good at acting and is no longer sure when she is playing a part – indeed, some others wonder if she is acting all the time. If she is alone, she gets bored and quickly looks for company again. She laughs and cries easily and is very sensitive to her surroundings. Although she has many boyfriends and would like to get married eventually, she finds it hard to choose between them. The young men that interest her most are usually unreliable, but the dependable boyfriend she always turns to in times of difficulty bores her at other times. She relies on other people a great deal and the thought that worries her most is that of being alone in the world.

The fussy type

Mr Eta is a senior official in a local government department. He prides himself on his conscientiousness and reliability. He has never been late for work in 30 years and people say that they might as well set their watches by his arrival time as he is more punctual than any clock. He likes everything to run according to a set routine and his department runs like clockwork. He does not like change, so, if he is asked to take on an entirely new problem, he is put out at first because he has no rules to follow. He dresses soberly and conventionally and is formal in his social relationships. Looking ahead is his watchword and he likes to plan as far into the future as possible so that it is predictable. In his spare time, he collects stamps and coins, and these are beautifully ordered and presented. After work each day, he spends 35 minutes sorting and resorting these, then feels completely at peace with the world. Modern society he detests because it appears to have lost contact with order and discipline, and he tries to introduce these qualities into all aspects of his life and work. He lives in a neat house in a quiet suburb and has respectable neighbours who share his views. His garden is exceptionally well looked after, although some feel he tries too hard to make his lawn look like a bowling green and his impeccable display of bedding plants – wallflowers in the spring, petunias and marigolds in the summer – might sometimes be changed for something new.

Using what we've found out

These descriptions of personality types are too short to get anything more than a glimpse of the kinds of people they represent, and whole books could be written about each of them. Nevertheless, I think that you should have little difficulty in identifying people you know in one or more of the descriptions and may recognize yourself in the example of the personality type you obtained from the questionnaire. You may have some difficulty in accepting the picture of yourself painted by the example, but, remember, each one is a stereotype. The people of this world cannot be put into only seven groups, but they share many characteristics. You should at least recognize some aspects of yourself in one of the types I have described. Once you have decided on the personality type attributed to you by the questionnaire, stick to it, even if the fit is far from perfect, because this will be needed in the exercise we are carrying out later.

How is stress related to these personality types? The most impressive differences are found between the driving, successful (Ms Alpha) and placid, easy-going personalities (Mr Beta). Research in the United States over many years has shown that the Alphas (the Mr more than the Ms) of this world are two to five times more likely than the Mr Betas to suffer heart disease. If we accept that heart disease can be the result of prolonged, harmful stress, it is easy to see how driving, aggressive, successful people are likely to be stressed. They go around looking for challenges and changes that create more demands on mind and body. They never relax and, even when they have achieved one target in life, they set themselves another – usually it is even more demanding. What is unfortunate is that each success in life encourages them to strive still harder. One way in which our society creates unnecessary stress is by excessively praising success in every walk of life, and making out that if you are not a success you must automatically be a failure.

Most advertising slogans shout at you to become successful or else perish in mediocrity. 'You too can be successful at work and with the opposite sex; you too can be a successful tycoon, you too can have a marvellous memory and wow your friends' and so it goes on. Promises are made to improve your self-confidence, appearance and even change the person you are into someone quite different, someone you want to be. (One person I know has a different extension of himself to accommodate all these people, but he has other problems.) However, if you stop to think about these claims, you will realize that they cannot be true. If it was really so easy to achieve these aims, then everyone would be successful and the world would be full of successful clones who would be so predictable that they would be utterly boring. In the words of W. S. Gilbert, 'If everyone is somebody, then no one's anybody.' All success comes from competition and there can only be a few winners. Where our society has a lot to answer for is in its adulation of the winner. Once he has won, he has to go on winning and, if he falters in the slightest, he is abandoned as a failure. Our personalities are partly moulded by the environment in which we live and, although our driving successful Alphas may destroy themselves, they are encouraged to do so by society. They rise to the top of national and multinational organizations, make them more efficient so that they make bigger profits. More money can be invested to make the organization bigger so it can employ more people and produce more. This is the message of capitalism, and global capitalism in particular. By producing more, we sell more as standards of living are raised and every country becomes more prosperous. It sounds so good that many people believe this to be true.

So, although you probably read the description of Ms Alpha with distaste and recognized none of her characteristics in you, she is the most favoured personality type in our Western society. I am sure that you have wished you were more like her at some time in your life – particularly when you have come across a problem and not had the stamina or will to overcome it. Much of our lives are governed by Alpha principles laid down by society. The Peter principle, named after a Canadian who first described it, is that people at work are promoted until they reach the level of their own incompetence. To begin with, they are in junior, low-paid posts, but, as they master these, they are promoted to senior ones. As each new post is tackled and overcome, new horizons beckon until, at last, a post is attained that is just too much for them to cope with. This is the peak of occupational success and obviously varies from person to person. Unfortunately, this post is often the most stressful of them all, because it makes demands on us that cannot be compensated for. We are playing the success–stress game without realizing it.

When we read about business executives with ulcers, heart disease, high blood pressure and other diseases exacerbated by stress we naturally think that their jobs are the prime cause of their troubles. This, though, is far too simple an explanation. We select the driving, successful personalities for the important executive posts because they are the only ones who can cope with them. Of course, once they are in such posts their personalities are allowed full expression and stress is increased. Unfortunately, too many jobs require the same qualities of energy, drive, competitiveness, intense self-discipline and desire to succeed. Although this demand seems to be creating more Alphas in our midst – evidence suggests there are more in America than in the UK – far too many of us are encouraged to believe that we have these qualities when, in fact, we lack them. If we take such jobs, we are like square pegs in round holes – stress and conflict increase and we suffer unnecessarily. So, do not give in too readily to demands that you should 'make a success of your life' and take on a lifestyle that is quite alien to you.

Matching your personality to your life

To keep harmful stress to a minimum, your personality needs to be matched to your lifestyle. We just need to look at the way our different personality types cope with the same external situations to realize why stress affects each of us in a different way. Imagine asking each of our seven personalities to make a speech on a subject of his or her choice to a group of people. Ms Alpha would have no problem with public speaking and produce an impressive, driving and polished speech, but it would have to be fitted in with many other demands on her time. Mr Beta would probably not prepare a speech at all and instead give a fireside chat. Miss Gamma would be thrown into a panic at the thought of public speaking and do her utmost to get out of the task, as would Mr Epsilon who would hate to talk to so many strangers. On the other hand, Miss Zeta and Mr Delta would positively enjoy the occasion as it would add sparkle and novelty to the day. Mr Eta would take the occasion seriously and prepare his speech with great care, possibly practising in front of a mirror beforehand to make sure he looked and sounded the part. While the exercise of standing up in public and talking in a way that makes reasonable sense is bound to have some stressful elements, the main difference between those who do not mind public speaking and those who are troubled by it is that the latter are stressed for a long time before, and sometimes after, the speaking. If we are asked to recall the most nerve-racking part of speaking in public, most of us would pick the time immediately before we start speaking. This is the time when our mouths feel dry, our voices croak, our legs feel like jelly and we wish we were a hundred miles away. The thought of feeling like this would make Miss Gamma refuse to do the talk as she would worry for weeks in advance and probably be paralysed by fright when the time came for the speech. While Mr Beta might be mildly stressed for 20 minutes during his talk, Miss Gamma would be afflicted by major stress for many weeks.

Another reason for stress affecting each of us differently is that the change it produces in us varies from one person to another. Swimming a long distance is no problem for an experienced swimmer, but for those who are unfit and rarely swim it is an ordeal that leaves them exhausted for the rest of the day. The stress of more ordinary changes also shows similar variations. If each of our personality types was required to move house, there would be different kinds of stress experienced. Mr Delta is so used to moving that he can do it while half asleep. Mr Epsilon and Mr Eta tend to stay in the same place whenever they have the choice. Of course, personality matches with behaviour, as the types who hate change keep it to a minimum, but it means that those who dislike a particular stress have the least experience of dealing with it.

Although we have remarkable abilities to overcome problems and adapt to strange situations, we must not assume that we are superhuman. We may like or dislike our basic personalities, but we cannot ignore them. It also used to be thought that they did not change to a significant degree, but now we know that, over many years, personality does change (Seivewright, et al., 2002). Mr Delta and Miss Zeta tend to become less strong in their personality attributes over time, but Mr Eta, Miss Gamma and Mr Epsilon may find their characteristics becoming stronger. Therapies to change matters are also available, but only Miss Zeta should join the queue for these because there is insufficient evidence that they are effective for the other types.

Those who like to plan people's lives sometimes have visions of a future when personality can be changed to order. Just imagine what a terrible world that would be. We might choose to be super-efficient successful people such as Ms Alpha, but, if there is no one to control or supervise, we will have a country of prime ministers with no people to govern. If the power to change personality fell into the hands of a dictator, we could be programmed to be dull, obedient slaves with no independent thoughts or actions. No, the variation in personality is too precious to be thrown away. Coming to terms with ourselves and accepting our strengths and weaknesses honestly is a necessary prelude to living with stress. This is not an easy task. 'O wad some Pow'r the giftie gie us, to see oursels as others see us!', wrote Robert Burns ('To a Louse'). Most of us do not have that power, but at least we can listen to what others have to say. Once we have accepted our personalities – warts and all – we can plan our lives in a more sensible way.

4

How to recognize harmful stress

In this part of the book I shall be describing different ways to treat harmful stress. Harmful stress, which includes distress and strain, has no advantages and should be kept to a minimum, if not eliminated altogether. Rather than describe each of the ways of treating stress in neat little chapters, I want you to come with me on a voyage of discovery. It is like one of the mystery tours beloved of coach operators where the passengers have no idea of their destination when they board the bus. In this case, however, I want each reader to be a driver. The route will be decided by your personalities. Each personality type will take a different route, but I would like to think that you will end up at destinations that have one thing in common: they are free from harmful stress. The reason for choosing this approach, which means that from now onwards you could read the rest of the book in any order, is our old chestnut, the individuality of stress. It is impossible to say that any one way of coping with stress is better than any other because not only do the causes differ, but also the people who show the effects of stress.

If you have any of the symptoms we have discussed in earlier chapters, the question you need to ask is simply this – 'Are my symptoms getting better or worse?' If they are getting worse, your stress is not doing you any good and may be doing you harm. Unfortunately, no one can put a timescale on stress, but, in general, we are talking about unpleasant feelings that have lasted for weeks or months when we refer to harmful stress. Also, if they are getting worse but have only lasted a day or so, you can assume for the time being that they are healthy.

When it comes to distinguishing between mental stress and the normal ups and downs of life, we are in difficult territory. In the last resort, each individual has to decide where that dividing line is. Some people can be under stress even though everything in their lives is satisfactory, at least in a material way. They have jobs that are interesting and in which they can go at their own pace, they are happily married with delightful children and are physically fit. Not a cloud seems to be visible in their personal skies, yet they can have all the symptoms of stress. Why? The reason is that their lives have no meaning. Nothing they do seems to matter and so they are troubled. Even if there is no obvious explanation for your feelings of dissatisfaction, they can still be due to stress.

Detecting silent, harmful stress is not an exercise you can easily do alone. Although you should be able to appreciate the symptoms of stress, you put a mental block on your awareness and pretend that nothing is wrong. True, others may be constantly telling you to calm down and take less responsibility or may be suffering as a result of your response to stress, but you ignore them. I pointed out earlier that only you can judge the intensity of your own feelings, but others are in a better position to judge how they affect those around you. You might not be aware of any feelings of stress and only show it by making a misery of other people's lives. So, if people are yearning for a time in the past when you were a nicer person to live with, or work for, or if you find that your friends are melting away and no longer seeking your company, perhaps you should think if it is you rather than they that have changed. The suspicious Epsilons among you will find such an admission very difficult. It is surprising how often people can look back at times in their lives when they behaved out of character and be amazed that they failed to recognize the problems that now are transparently clear. You can avoid this by listening with more attention to the comments of people you respect and not just dismissing them as ignorant criticisms.

Personality journeys

I have chosen to separate your personalities in the routes you take through this book, because each type has a different susceptibility to stress. The ambitious Alphas are particularly liable to succumb to the physical diseases of stress – peptic ulcers, coronary heart disease, migraine and high blood pressure. People in this group are in control of their emotions and mental stress is much less common. Feelings of anger, irritability, nervousness and depression are sometimes noticed but are quickly suppressed. They get in the way of success and progress and can be forgotten. The stress therefore has its main impact on the body. Our worrying Gammas are much more likely to suffer mental stress. The reactions of the sympathetic nervous system that we all feel occasionally happen so frequently with them that they seem to dominate their lives. These people are much less likely to develop the physical diseases of stress, although they do so more often than the placid Betas. It may be an oversimplification, but it appears that if stress can be expressed outwardly in the form of mental disturbance, it is less likely to turn inwards and affect the body.

Placid types show the least harmful stress. This is predictable, because they are seekers of stability, not of change, and happiest when few demands are made on them. They experience less stress in all its forms, both healthy and harmful, than the other types and so suffer much less from its ill effects. The other personality types have less clear-cut relationships with stress, but there still are differences between them. The conscientious Etas who like to have the whole of their lives organized in advance suffer stress if they are repeatedly asked to adjust to changes that are beyond their control. Although they can show both mental and bodily stress, they tend towards the latter. Their high principles and strong sense of duty often lead to them experiencing greater stress than other types of personality as they will tolerate the intolerable for much longer.

The carefree Deltas are closest to the placid Betas and have a much lower predisposition to harmful stress. However, their need for variety and excitement leads them into many potentially harmful situations that others would not contemplate. Our illustration of Mr Delta described a man who liked parachute jumping, but this is only one example of sought-after stress. Deltas are more likely to have accidents because they take risks in all areas of life. They drive fast and recklessly and often seek out danger. They lack foresight and do things that fulfil their need for excitement because of the risks involved. It is unfortunate that they can only reach the extreme levels of excitement they crave by taking risks and courting disaster. The high wire artiste who performs incredible feats of agility at dizzying heights above the ground creates much more excitement for himself and his audience if he does not use a safety net. The Delta types are unwilling to derive all their excitement in the form of passive spectacle – at the circus, race track, football field or boxing ring – and prefer to be actively involved.

The dependent Zetas and suspicious Epsilons are more likely to suffer the mental consequences of harmful stress, but under quite different circumstances. Zetas do not like being alone and any prolonged isolation will be highly unpleasant for them. They express their feelings readily – almost too readily for some people who wonder if they are exaggerated at times – and are likely to respond to the ups and downs of life with appropriate displays of emotion. The Epsilons, on the other hand, prefer to be alone and are most distressed when they are forced to rub shoulders with many people, particularly when there is no opportunity to avoid them. This stress, which is actively desired by the Zetas, is harmful to the Epsilons because it reinforces their worries and suspicions and shows in both the mental and physical spheres. Such people prefer having a few people around them whom they can trust absolutely – the rest of humanity are potential enemies.

Although most of the ingredients of a problem likely to produce harmful stress are unique, there is an important contribution from personality. I emphasize again that we cannot change personality, so simple solutions to stress are just not realistic. Making everybody adopt the lifestyle of the placid Betas in our midst on the grounds that it would reduce stress would be quite wrong. This lifestyle would be incompatible with all the other personality types and therefore produce a host of new stresses. We noted earlier that everyone has an optimum level of stress at which they are most happy, and there are great differences in these levels between our personality types. Harmful stress can result if the level of stimulation becomes too low as well as too high.

Our personality types vary in terms of the risk of suffering harmful stress and the ways in which it is usually shown. These are summarized below so that you can see at a glance how your own personality type fares.

Type of personality	Risk of harmful stress	Type of harmful stress
Ambitious	Very high	Physical
Placid	Very low	Physical
Worrying	Very high	Mental
Carefree	Low	Physical
Suspicious	Moderate	Mental and physical
Dependent	Moderate	Mental
Fussy	Moderate	Physical

We can now start our mystery tour. The first stage is easy and most of us will continue on the same route. The only ones who are going to be diverted are the anxious worrying types of personality we came across in the last chapter. If you are like Miss Gamma, who has always been highly anxious, I would like you to move straight on to Chapter 6. I emphasize that here I am only referring to people who have tended to be nervous all their lives and can never remember being any different. Others may have a very good reason for feeling anxious, but, at some time in the past, before they were put under stress, they were not nervous. Nobody is under constant stress from the moment they are born to the time they die, so, if you cannot recollect being calm and relaxed at any time in your life, you must be a Gamma-type personality. There is some evidence that this personality type runs in families, so if you feel you are in this category I would not be surprised if one or more of your close relatives felt similarly.

All other personality types should continue to Chapter 5, no matter what type of stress you have been under and how long it has lasted. You will be going on your separate ways in due course, so do not be concerned.

5

Survival of the fittest

You probably recognize this expression. It was first used to describe Charles Darwin's theory of evolution – a theory proposed nearly 150 years ago. Darwin suggested that all living things developed from a common ancestor by a gradual process taking millions of years. Chance variations from one generation to the next accounted for all the differences in the animal and plant kingdoms. Most of these variations were of no long-term value and so the species died out – the most famous examples are the dinosaurs – but some of the changes were very useful because they made the animal or plant better suited to its surroundings. So they thrived and multiplied at the expense of other species. Such a series of chance variations, according to the theory, led to the emergence of the most successful species of them all – human beings. Humans are successful because of our superior intelligence. This not only helps us to defeat competitors, but gives us the power to change and control our living conditions in a way granted to no other species, so that we are even better suited to our surroundings. So the phrase 'survival of the fittest' is well suited to human beings. The weak go to the wall and the strong survive.

Evolution and stress

What has this got to do with stress? A great deal. We go through exactly the same process in our daily lives. When we come across a problem, we have two choices: we can solve or overcome it or we can avoid it. Better still, we organize a niche for ourselves in life that is so well suited to us that we do not come across serious problems at all. This is the ultimate aim of the treatment called nidotherapy that we will come across in Chapter 11. Which choice we make depends a great deal on our personalities. The driving, successful type – the Alphas we came across earlier – are always looking for new heights to scale, new problems to solve, and are more concerned about changing their surroundings than living in harmony with them. These are the people who are most prone to diseases stemming from stress because they deliberately put themselves under pressure and

49

are only happy when they are in the thick of things. If you are this type of personality, you are not going to change this pattern of living because it would be completely out of character. Your best policy is to concentrate on controlling the harmful effects of stress by means of one of the techniques described in the next chapter. You can move straight on to Chapter 6 now if you wish.

Of course this is not the best way of dealing with stress because you are only lessening the stress rather than removing it. There are many others who may on the surface be like the driving Alpha types, but their basic personalities are quite different. They are forced by outside pressures to drive themselves harder than they would like; they are controlled by, rather than controlling, their lives. The trouble is that the more successful they are the more the pressures crowd in. Almost every day we can pick up a newspaper and read that some household name – a politician, pop star, sports celebrity or entertainer – has succumbed to stress in one form or another. Yet another overdose has been taken or the star's personal physician has advised complete rest because of 'severe strain' or the entertainer has broken down on stage. Once carried away by the system of success it is difficult to escape, except through illness.

Success so often means keeping up an image, which really means living a lie. The face the public sees is not your real face. It is a plastic face fashioned by the publicists, all of whom grow fat on your success while it destroys you. Perhaps the best people to cope with this type of stress are those who, from birth onwards, are in the public eye, such as members of the Royal Family. However, recent events have shown that even these people are far from immune. At least if you spend all your years in the glare of publicity you are more likely to adapt to the pressures that it brings. For others who have the misfortune to have fame thrust on them, the important thing is to keep your public and private faces as natural as possible. Even the best actor sometimes has an off day and the strain of a role that goes against your true self will eventually grind you down.

You may feel that I am painting too gloomy a picture of success. My concern is with uncontrolled success in any part of life – be it at work, leisure or in relationships with others. We all need an element of success in life to maintain our self-esteem and, provided it is not exploited too much, this can bring rewards without harmful stress. We also need to be reminded that failure can also be very stressful. The failure of the jilted lover, the bankrupt tycoon or the unsuccessful examination candidate is so often stressful because our pride is hurt. Sometimes the blow is too hard to bear and suicide is seen as the only way out of the conflict.

The highest rate of suicide this century was not, as you might expect, during the horrifying stresses of war, but in peacetime, during the Great Depression (a very apt name) following the economic collapse in 1929. Those who were the most well off had more to lose and many committed suicide rather than face the indignity of abandoning their former way of life. They all felt some personal responsibility for their financial ruin even when it was caused by factors beyond their control. When similar destruction to property and living standards was caused by the Blitz in World War II, the people who suffered felt no personal responsibility for their plight. Suicide fell to the lowest level for many years, but the stress still wreaked its damage and the number of peptic ulcers shot up alarmingly.

In our present affluent society, we seldom come across such severe stresses, ones that are quite beyond our control. As noted earlier, we have a choice of actions. Of course, the very fact of having a choice can produce its own share of stress, as often we cannot decide between conflicting interests. For example, many have commented on the eerie calm that comes over men sentenced to death in the minutes before their execution, but of course at this time there is no personal choice left and the stress is much less than earlier, when perhaps they entertained some hope of reprieve.

In making a choice, it is helpful to bear in mind what we said earlier about the survival of the fittest. The best choice is the one that leads to the best match between you and your surroundings. When Darwin first proposed his theory, he used the phrase 'survival of the adapted' and only later was 'adapted' changed to 'fittest', and then only as a catchy title. Let us see exactly what Darwin said (*On the Origin of Species*, 1859):

> As the individuals of the same species come in all respects into the closest competition with each other, the struggle will generally be most severe between them. On the other hand the struggle will often be severe between beings remote in the scale of nature. The slightest advantage in certain individuals, at any age or during any season, over those with which they come into competition, or better adaptation in however slight a degree to the surrounding physical conditions, will, in the long run, turn the balance.

You will note that Darwin recognizes the merit of adaptation over naked struggle – the latter being a prominent, but limited, way to demonstrate advantage. 'Adapted' is a better word than 'fittest' because it includes all the ways in which you can cope with the problems of stress, while 'fittest' suggests that only drive and aggression will succeed. It is only when you have adapted to the changes at the heart of stress that you can say you have overcome it.

So, successful adaptation is the best 'cure' for your stress. Of course it is not a 'cure' in the real sense because you have removed the cause rather than treated the disease. Although on the surface this appears less glamorous than curing your stress with some special treatment, it is much better because, if it is done properly, the stress will not come back. However, like most things in life, the best approach is the one needing the most work. It is much easier to pretend that stress-related disease is not a personal problem but a medical one because this means you can absolve yourself from responsibility. If the treatment you receive fails in any way, you can blame others instead of yourself and, if it succeeds, you have been told what to do rather than working out the solution for yourself. There are no easy answers to the problems caused by stress as each personal stress has unique qualities and the ideal treatment is also unique, carefully fashioned for that problem alone.

Taking personality into account

It is still possible to give guidance on how to go about adapting to harmful stress. We have to remember that, to adjust successfully, we must bear our basic personalities in mind. Otherwise, we can make what appears to be a marvellous adjustment at first, but, if this conflicts with the habitual behaviour of our basic personalities, it will soon rebound on us. The driving, ambitious type who decides to opt out of his job as head of an international combine and go back to nature in a remote wilderness may at first be relieved at disgorging his stressful lifestyle. However, before long, his competitive urges will be rekindled and he will only be happy if he can organize the rural community in the same way as he did his former company.

There is clear evidence of this from experience, suggesting the conclusion 'once a tycoon, always a tycoon'. Tycoon Alpha when transplanted from the City of London to the north of Scotland decides to do a little local craft work to keep busy. Only a short time later, though, our tycoon will see the opportunities for mass production and improved sales by advertising and soon the crofting community is another big business. (This is the second opportunity for any driving ambitious personalities who are still with us to move on to Chapter 6.)

We so often let harmful stress get out of control because of blind spots in our make-up that stop us from seeing the obvious solution. Let us look at some typical examples of this among the personality types we came across earlier.

Mr Beta, you will recall, is placid, good-natured and perhaps a little lazy. In general, he is protected from stress, but, like many placid people, he enjoys food. Unfortunately, people who enjoy food and do not take a great deal of exercise are liable to eat more than their bodies need. So, Mr Beta puts on weight. He does not admit to himself that he eats too much or is overweight, but he agrees with his close friends that he has 'a weight problem' (this satisfies the notion that someone else may help in solving it). He wonders whether or not this might be something to do with his glands and visits the doctor, who examines him and tells him bluntly that he is overweight and so must be eating too much. Mr Beta cannot believe this. He never eats between meals and, although he enjoys his food, he has never been greedy.

When it is pointed out that his meals are three times bigger than those of other members of his family and his penchant for cakes and buns makes it more likely for him to put on weight, he protests how little food they contain because they are light and full of air. If he takes no notice and stays overweight, he will become tired easily, feel depressed because he is not able to do as much as he used to and have many arthritic aches and pains. These symptoms would all be due to him carrying round a body that is 50 per cent heavier than his frame is built for. It may take him many months to accept the simple fact that he is eating too much and that fat cannot come out of thin air.

One reason for his finding this so difficult is that eating plays such an important part in his life. He is hospitable, sociable and generous and food is involved in many of his activities. Once food is established as one of the good things in life, it is very difficult to accept that it can do harm. However, if he can come to terms with his problem and realize that it can be overcome by sticking to a proper weight loss plan, either as a result of his own efforts or with the assistance of an organization such as Weight Watchers, and if losing weight can be achieved without resorting to pills or other medical forms of treatment, it is likely to be successful in the long run.

Mr Epsilon and other suspicious personality types usually produce different stress problems. In fact, they are frequently thin and underweight. In days of old, they might have employed food tasters to test each meal and make sure that it was not poisoned! The niche that suits Mr Epsilon is a small one and he quickly becomes stressed if he moves out of it. For instance, the headteacher of his school feels that Mr Epsilon's many years of devoted service to teaching should be rewarded by making him deputy headteacher. This is accepted gratefully by Mr Epsilon, who is glad that his true worth has been recognized. His duties involve much less teaching and more tasks such as organizing the school curriculum. When taken away from the children, with whom he feels secure, Mr Epsilon becomes more suspicious. He spends most of his time with other teachers, discussing and coordinating their work. Occasionally, and inevitably with this type of work, there are minor disagreements. Mr Epsilon inflates these into major crises in his own mind and every criticism is seen as a personal attack. He feels the other staff are all against him and plotting his downfall. He cannot concentrate on his work and it naturally suffers. I need not go any further as you can predict the consequences if the stress is not removed. Mr Epsilon should never have accepted, or even have been offered, the deputy headteacher post. He should be rapidly restored to his previous position or moved to a similar one in another school if the damage to his relationships has gone too far.

Those of us who become heavily involved in relationships or need people to the extent of depending on them, such as Miss Zeta, are likely to come across harmful stress in these relationships. Such people need attention and variety in life, but are troubled by insecurity. So, Miss Zeta might be very tempted to commit herself and move in with her dependable boyfriend – one of the few signs of constancy in her life. This may be the right course, but is not necessarily an answer to her uncertainty.

If he is interested in settling down and leading a more predictable life, conflict lies ahead. Miss Zeta is not quite sure what she wants and, although she is unsettled and uncertain about herself, she is attracted to the idea that all her options are still open and the world, not a small, cosy niche, is her oyster.

The change to a quieter life, particularly if it is forced by circumstances, may be too great for her to bear. As it conflicts with her personality, she may never adapt to it (although, as we said earlier, this will become easier with age and adaptation could come later). The temptation to keep her risky but exciting former lifestyle will be strong and is bound to conflict with the expectations of her more sober partner. She may not even be certain of her sexual orientation and forcing her life into a clearly heterosexual mode may make her realize that the close relationships she had with some of her modelling colleagues were more satisfying than this one.

Of course, there are many reasons for relationships not working out and it would be wrong to blame them all on personality clashes. In Miss Zeta's case, the solution is likely to involve acceptance – by both her and those around her (there is a terrible expression 'significant others' used to describe these people) – that she is uncertain and cannot be forced into situations that deny the presence of this uncertainty. No, she is not a home-loving domesticated dutiful wife or partner, who is happy to stay on her own all day and spend quiet evenings with her husband. Her personality demands variety. She needs her independence and freedom and forcing her to give up either of these will promote stress.

By now you will be getting into the swing of things and could probably predict the changes that would lead to harmful stress for the carefree Mr Delta. This personality type likes variety, is impulsive, sometimes a little childish and rather vain. Because Mr Delta has little foresight and is prone to flattery, it is easy to see how success could turn sour on him. Suppose a national broadcasting company was to discover hidden talents in him and make him a DJ with his own show or set him up to front a chat show. He would become instantly popular (in this day and age such an outcome is absolutely predictable), but, instead of putting this into perspective, he would be convinced that he really was a great guy. His life would lose all semblance of control. He would become involved in complicated personal relationships with his female fans, his working and leisure time would be a whirl of continual change with no time for reflection and he would overreach himself as vanity quickly replaced common sense. The cycle of success would get out of hand and the stress would finally surface as drug use or an overdose, alcoholism or, the ultimate humiliation, a breakdown while on air. Dealing with this type of stress in Mr Delta would be a difficult problem. He and success do not mix and, if he were unfortunate enough to become a star, his best hope would be to have a good agent who would protect him from the publicity that would otherwise destroy him.

The anxious worrying types will not be reading this chapter, so we can exclude an example of Miss Gamma under stress. Unfortunately, virtually every change that is in any way out of the ordinary is going to have damaging effects on her. So, we move on to our final type – fussy Mr Eta. As noted earlier, this type is highly organized and tries to keep change to a minimum by adjusting to it in advance. However, many changes are beyond his control. He likes his peace and quiet and, although he can tolerate a fair amount of bustle and activity, it becomes disturbing if it interferes with his routines. If his quiet house and garden were to change from being a desirable residential area because it was in the flight path of an airport, he would begin to have problems. The continual roar of aircraft overhead and the increased bustle of activity around his home would be disturbing, although he would be less inclined to move house than other personality types because of his dislike of change. However, if the excessive noise and activity increased he would lose control. We need to remind ourselves that excessive noise and overcrowding are not natural to us and, although we may often choose to live in a city because it is close to our work and has a better range of shopping, entertainment and other facilities than the country, it is far from being our ideal surroundings.

Stress compensation is better than stress treatment

People are social beings and live best in groups, but not when they are very large. When there are too many people packed into a small space, it becomes stressful for everybody. When other animals are overcrowded in this way, they run out of food and large numbers leave the group, even when the alternatives are far from attractive. You have probably heard of the lemming – a small animal, rather like a vole, that responds to overcrowding by mass emigration. Thousands of lemmings will file into the sea from an overcrowded island, only a few surviving to reach new land. We do not have the same degree of sensitivity to overcrowding, but it does have effects on us. Unfortunately, the drift to the cities is continuing in almost all countries of the world. As stress follows change and the amount and speed of change is so much greater in cities than the countryside, all the problems of stress are greater in cities. Those who live in small

56

towns or rural surroundings will live, on the average, nearly five years longer than those in cities, where there are also more instances of the diseases of harmful stress. Although Mr Eta would be disinclined to make a move because of his unwillingness to make big changes in his life, he would suffer if he decided to stay, unless he could band together with like-minded residents and persuade the authorities that the proposed changes are detrimental to their quality of life and should be abandoned or channelled elsewhere.

Obviously we could go on indefinitely conjuring up scenes from the lives of these personalities that would be unpleasantly stressful for some and have no effect on others, but I hope the general message is clear from the examples we have looked at here. The ideal way to deal with harmful stress is to neutralize it in exactly the same way that healthy stress is overcome. The resources needed to cancel our stress are often considerable and it may be a long haul. However, we often fail to overcome stress properly because we adopt old ways of dealing with it. Most of the time, our minds run along well-ordered grooves like the wheels of a tram and this protects us from a lot of unnecessary stress. However, harmful stress only develops when these grooves are no longer right for us and we have to make new ones. This means thinking, and thinking means hard work. Until we recognize the problem, though, we will never find the solution. When we recognize the symptoms of stress, it is much easier to rush off and try one of the treatments for stress described in later chapters than it is to ponder a little and work out why we feel as we do. It is also much more difficult to remove the problem than to treat the symptoms directly. All the pressures are on us to take the easy way out and try the latest treatment for stress. We shall find that they are not as impressive as they appear to be and can never cure stress. This needs repeating, particularly as we are constantly being assailed by the latest and best of anti-stress treatments, which so often claim to cure, but never can.

In removing harmful stress, we come back time and time again to the paramount importance of balancing our internal needs with the pressures from outside. So many of us live lives today that are highly specialized because society demands experts in everything. However, a balanced society in which every member has a specialized role produces a lot of highly unbalanced individuals. The professor who is trained to teach, write and develop new knowledge is not encouraged to treat his illnesses, mend his plumbing when it springs a leak or service his own car. All these jobs are done by other experts who require special training, so that life becomes chopped up by hundreds of demarcation lines, each special task needing a solution from someone other than ourselves. However, the professor is not just a walking brain, much as society may like him to be, and his body and mind require the same balance of activities as the rest of humanity.

In talking about the survival of the adapted in our present age, we should not just try to achieve the somewhat artificial goals set by society, but set targets for ourselves. Although, as we have seen, people have different goals and require different levels of stress to keep in balance, they all have certain basic needs. 'Do you feel fit?' is perhaps the simplest way of deciding whether you are under harmful stress or have any form of illness. Fitness includes both physical and mental wellbeing and can only be attained by proper use of our bodies and minds. If you never take any exercise apart from walking to the local shops or pushing the vacuum cleaner over the floor you cannot be physically fit. You will feel so much better if you take more exercise. Of course, if you have spent many years being underactive and overweight, some damage may already have been done, so you would be advised not to suddenly do strenuous activities. Every winter there is a disquieting number of deaths following heavy snowfalls when people have to dig the snow away from around their cars. For those unfamiliar with exercise the result is often a heart attack with fatal consequences. Just in the same way that a mind which is never asked to think will produce tension and anxiety when forced to work out a problem, a body that is never exercised will fail when asked to take on a physical task. This is not to say that we should all be Tarzans and Janes, swinging through the trees in a self-indulgent display of muscular prowess, but Western society in general is physically unfit and needs to be reminded that this is so. Our ancestors recognized the value of keeping a balance between work, rest and play, and although at times they were a little rigid in the application of their philosophy, we could do with a dose of it nowadays.

If you think that you are suffering from harmful stress, I would like to think that, after finishing this chapter, you will know what is causing it and already have some idea as to how you are going to rid yourself of it. The most successful among you will not need any of the special aids described later because you will be able to put yourselves back into balance by means of your own efforts. This does not mean that success will come immediately. Often you may be inhibited from taking the right corrective action because, in the short term, it appears to be wrong. Nobody likes to stop eating when they feel hungry or ask for demotion, because it means a big drop in income, but if you never take the first step, you will be stuck indefinitely. You will also have realized from this chapter that how others have coped with their stresses may be quite irrelevant to your problem, and any advice you take should be from people you know well and whose judgement you respect. In any case, you are going to have to make the final decision in the end, no matter how many people advise you on the way.

If you think you have learnt nothing from this chapter and cannot wait to read on for some straight talk about treating stress directly, then by all means move on. However, such a reaction implies that you already know why you are suffering from stress but have done nothing to remove it. This may be true, but we tend to assume that it is true when change is possible. As we live in a world of change, there is no reason for you to be exempt. So, why wait for a crisis to show you how to overcome your stress? If you are right in fully appreciating why you are suffering, it is ridiculous to accept a second-best treatment if you have any possibility of removing or lessening the cause. I am confident that all the placid Betas among you will be able to do this successfully, but, first of all, read Chapter 10. Some others of you will also be able to conquer your stress without any special help, but all the rest should come with me to Chapter 6.

6
Self-control

Before we go into detail about how to control harmful stress through our own efforts, we should recap the progress we have made so far. We are assuming that you cannot banish stress from your lives either because you are such a worrying type that everything is stressful or you cannot find the cause of your stress or you know the cause only too clearly but can do nothing about removing it. Whatever the reason, the stress is harmful because it is with you continuously. The first part of treatment is to break into this cycle where the sympathetic nervous system and other hormones of stress have a completely free hand and replace it with relaxation. Then, you will no longer feel anxious and worried, your muscles will no longer be tense and your heart and breathing rate will slow to a regular resting level. When you are well, you have no problem relaxing, but when you are under continual stress, a lot of work is needed to earn a few moments of calm.

Relaxation techniques

There are relaxation techniques that will help to make these moments last longer. Read and follow the instructions below and you will understand the principles behind these techniques. It needs practice before you can relax fully at will and it is a good idea to start when you are already fairly relaxed. So, for maximum effect, follow the instructions after you have had a hot bath or feel tired after a hard day of physical work.

Relaxing the body

Find a comfortable, supportive chair or lie on your bed or the floor, if it is warm and comfortable – you could spread out a blanket, large towel or exercise or camping mat to cushion you.

First, tense the muscles of your right hand by making a fist. Hold this tension for half a minute. If you feel your grip relaxing, tighten the fist still further. Slowly let the muscles relax and open out the hand and fingers. If your hand still feels tense, make a fist again. Slacken the fist gradually until the hand is quite floppy and relaxed.

Next, tense the arm and shoulder by bending the elbow and

bringing your hand up against your shoulder. Hold this position for at least a minute. Each muscle in your arm will feel tight and stiff, but, when you let them relax, they will feel heavier and more comfortable.

Now, tense and relax the muscles of your left hand and arm in the same way. It should take less time to relax this arm than the right arm, but continue until both arms are quite loose.

Move on next to the muscles of your neck and face. Exercise these muscles by raising and lowering your eyebrows, then gently putting your head right back and then bringing it down until your chin rests against your chest. Frown and relax your forehead alternately. Open and close your mouth and clench your teeth tightly together. Relax your jaw gradually and feel the tension go. Relax your neck and face so that all the muscles feel soft and smooth.

Expand your chest by taking a deep breath and holding it for a few seconds. Slowly breathe out and feel the chest muscles relax. Take another deep breath and continue breathing slowly and deeply, slowly and deeply. As you continue to breathe deeply, you will find it easier to relax all the muscles in your arms, chest, neck and face.

Now lift your right leg off the ground with the knee held straight, hold it up for a few seconds and then slowly lower it to the ground. Do the same with the left leg. Continue to do this until your legs feel so tired and heavy that they seem to sink into the ground when they are relaxed. As your legs become more relaxed, it is difficult to lift them up. Let them rest and feel the tension flowing away. Make sure that your feet, ankles and knees are completely relaxed as well before you let your legs rest completely.

Remember to continue your deep breathing while you relax further. Each time you breathe out, your muscles will relax a little more. Feel your body sinking down and getting heavier as you continue to breathe more deeply. Let your back and stomach muscles relax as you breathe and feel a warm glow of relaxation pass over your whole body. Every muscle should now feel relaxed and your mind completely calm. Close your eyes and let the feeling of relaxation take over. Try to open your eyes again. It is not worth the effort – your eyelids are too heavy and you do not want to disturb your relaxation. Outside pressures no longer trouble you and you feel cut off from the world. Nothing troubles you now you are completely calm, completely calm and relaxed.

You are bound to feel more relaxed now if you have followed these instructions to the letter, but you will have to practise the technique repeatedly before you feel the full benefit. Once you have mastered the technique, when you are already quite relaxed, you can move on and learn to relax when you are feeling tense and highly strung. Do not give up if at first the technique does not seem to be working. It takes time and application and often progress is made in fits and starts. Just when you feel that nothing has been achieved, the principles of the technique will suddenly click and you are on your way.

Eastern forms of relaxation

Because the art of relaxation is so sought after in our modern world, people have searched for bigger and better ways of achieving it. This is why there has been so much interest in yoga, transcendental meditation, t'ai chi and other Eastern philosophies. These are really concerned with a way of life and it is difficult to transpose them to our Western society without losing a great deal. Nevertheless, the relaxation techniques of these philosophies have been modified so that they can be practised on their own without necessarily taking on the religious beliefs and lifestyles they stem from. They are probably not so effective when used in isolation in this way but they have become increasingly popular over the last few years. I am not an expert on yoga and transcendental meditation – indeed, there are very few Western doctors who can claim to be – so I am not able to say which are the best forms of these treatments for stress. However, as far as relaxation is concerned, they are essentially more complicated forms of relaxation training.

For example, in transcendental meditation, which was founded by Maharishi Mahesh Yogi as a form of yoga, the aim is to concentrate on a thought in such a way that the thought itself disappears and the 'source of the thought' is reached. This difficult task can only be achieved by repeating a personal mantra – a ritual word that helps to drive other thoughts out of the mind during meditation. The meditator's concentration is directed entirely to this mental search, but, as it involves cutting out all other stimulation, it automatically leads to muscular relaxation, a slower heartbeat and deeper, more regular breathing. Other techniques involve more complicated rituals, but all achieve the same end if successful.

Special types of breathing are used in other forms of yoga. They involve filling the bottom of the lungs with air first, and the proportion of time spent breathing in and out is also carefully regulated.

Although it is possible to learn these techniques from books, most people find it more helpful to be taught them in a class. There is likely to be an evening or daytime yoga, t'ai chi or relaxation class near where you live and it does no harm to enquire and enrol. If you cannot make much headway with relaxation training alone, you could find yoga or t'ai chi quite a different proposition, so do not be disheartened. There are lots of variations on the different techniques and, although there is little to choose between them, it is best to stick to the same one rather than chopping and changing.

Once you become an expert, you can reach a degree of mind control that you never even suspected was possible. This will help you to blank your mind when the pressures of stress become too much. Just think of the advantages of having this ability. Instead of bringing all the troubles of the day home in the evening so that they prevent your attempts to relax, you can just switch off and forget them until the next morning. A lucky few can even learn the trick of switching off whenever they feel themselves becoming overstressed, so the man who feels nervous about giving a speech to a large audience goes to sleep for five minutes beforehand or someone like Miss Gamma, who cannot get off to sleep at night, carries out her relaxation exercises until she naturally drops off. However, this ideal degree of control is rare. It takes time to develop the ability to relax fully and many can only do it if they are in the right mood. It is most useful in putting a stop to stressful reactions that otherwise would reinforce themselves.

Hypnosis

Hypnosis can also be used to aid relaxation, but is sometimes made out to be a more powerful treatment than it really is. Under hypnosis, you are more suggestible and better able to respond to instructions to relax. This, of course, requires a hypnotist, who issues the instructions while you are in this suggestible frame of mind. In deep hypnosis, you can be so relaxed that you appear to be in a coma, but in fact you are still awake. Unfortunately, only a small number of people can be hypnotized to this degree. However, very few are completely unresponsive to hypnotic suggestion and it can certainly help you to relax further.

Although at first a hypnotist is likely to be needed to introduce us to the subject and illustrate the power of suggestion, later we can use the technique on ourselves by means of autohypnosis. If we feel relaxed when someone else is telling us to relax in a special way, there is no reason for us not do the telling ourselves. Some people, particularly the Miss Zetas who depend on others, may find this hard to believe, but there is nothing especially potent about hypnotists – their power lies in our belief in them and, to a lesser extent, in what the say. So, before long, you can achieve the same beneficial effects by repeating instructions to yourself or by listening to an audiotape.

A word of advice

There are many ways in which to bring the pleasures of relaxation into your life and I trust one of the ways I have described above will be successful for you. I suggest trying the method for relaxing the body (relaxation training) first of all, yoga or transcendental meditation second and only moving on to hypnosis if these fail. The main reason for suggesting this order is financial. Relaxation training and yoga are cheap to learn or even cost nothing at all, but hypnotists are expensive by comparison. Some have special skills at teaching relaxation and it is always better to choose one recommended by a friend rather than pick one at random.

If you are successful in controlling harmful stress by means of relaxation, you need go no further, although it may still be worth your while thinking about its cause. If the cause is still nagging away, you will continue to be troubled, even though you have an effective weapon to combat it at your disposal. There are other possible consequences. You may feel completely relaxed after trying the techniques, but the pain or ache you thought was due to stress is still there. If this happens with any symptom, whether it is physical or mental, it is reasonable to assume that it is not due to stress or, if it is, that it has gone beyond the realms of psychological control and is now part of an illness. Relaxation is often a good diagnostic test. If you have severe pain in your back and find it remains exactly the same even when you have systematically relaxed every muscle group in your body, then your pain is unlikely to be due to the tension of stress. Your muscles may be in spasm for many other reasons or the pain may really be an internal one that just feels as if it is on the surface even though it comes from inside the body. If you still suspect that your symptoms have a physical basis after you have got to this stage, then it is wise to see your doctor about it. For many, however, this could be the time you turn to reading a self-help book for the problem.

Self-help books and manuals

Here I may be preaching to the converted, because, by reading this book, you could be regarded as receiving self-help. However, I may be doing you an injustice. You might be reading this book because you find it interesting and stimulating or you are just curious or you have not the slightest idea what I am going on about and are still looking for a clue.

There are many advantages to self-help books, but also some disadvantages. The advantages (compared with other forms of treatment) are that they are cheap, allow you to go at your own pace and are easily accessible if you happen to forget that excellent piece of advice on page 33.

Other forms of communication are also competing with self-help books for attention. These include the Internet, where there are many opportunities for what have been called 'health-directed journeys', and computer-guided treatments, which are still in their infancy but seem to be very promising (Marks, 1999).

The main disadvantage of self-help approaches is that very few of them offer a dialogue with you, whose problems, no matter how similar they are in principle to others', are, nonetheless, unique. If you get stuck on a problem, then it is difficult to find a solution without calling someone for advice, and only the computer-aided treatments make any effort to provide this. Self-help approaches may also go badly wrong when, as it were, you don't get plugged in at the right point. Thus, for example, if you have a physical illness, such as hyperthyroidism (overactive thyroid) and spend many hours examining reasons for your apparent stress and its solutions, it is unlikely that you will achieve anything like the success you would gain from a visit to your doctor.

So, seeing your doctor may actually be the next stage for others in our mystery tour. This will apply particularly to those who make absolutely no progress with relaxation training or other techniques and angrily discard them as a waste of time. Our driving, ambitious and anxious, worrying personalities are most likely to be in this position and, if so, should move on to the next chapter. If you are one of these and make a little progress with relaxation but find that you cannot develop it further, then move ahead to Chapter 8. All other personalities should proceed as follows. Suspicious Epsilons and fussy Etas should also go to Chapter 8, but dependent Zetas and carefree Deltas should go to Chapter 9, although the Zetas would be well advised to remind themselves of the message in Chapter 4 again first. Placid types who still feel under stress should go to Chapter 10, but I think they will be few.

If you move on to any of the next four chapters, you are admitting to yourself that you cannot solve your harmful stress on your own or by using advice from friends and relatives. You are moving on to the unknown world in which experts, some real and some self-appointed, suggest treatment of some kind. Although it is a strange land, it is useful to know something of the terrain in advance so that misunderstanding can be kept to a minimum.

7

'Doctor, I can't go on like this'

The family doctor is the expert who is most frequently approached by people suffering from harmful stress. Many years ago, the doctor and the parish vicar or priest were the only ones who were available. Now there are alternatives, but a good doctor is still often in the best position to advise what is most appropriate.

Before going to see your doctor, it is useful to have some idea about how much he or she is likely to know about stress and stress-related illness. General practitioners (GPs), as their title implies, are trained in general aspects of medicine rather than concentrating on one speciality. This does not mean that they are all non-specialists as many illnesses, such as those of childhood, throat and chest infections, back pain, arthritis and migraine, are treated much more often by general practitioners than by any other doctors. Clearly, if these conditions become serious, others have to be brought in to manage them, but, generally, family doctors are very knowledge-able. As stress is a common cause of illness, your doctor is likely to have seen many people with problems similar to yours and may well be an expert on the subject. This said, the average GP in the United Kingdom has somewhere between 1,000 and 2,000 people on his or her list and even if each had the ability to deal with all the problems caused by stress, it would be quite impracticable to spend the time necessary to do so and cope with all the other demands of the practice as well.

The average consultation with a GP takes seven minutes and so no time should be wasted in getting your problem across. The other point worth emphasizing is that GPs are trained to identify physical illnesses more than mental problems. This is not because mental problems are uncommon in general practice – indeed, they make up nearly one in five of all consultations – but, at least until recently, treatment was much more effective for physical illnesses and it is important not to miss diagnosing something treatable.

Harmful stress can be present in many forms, so it is no good simply saying to the doctor that you are suffering from stress. That is about as informative as saying that you feel ill. Say what your symptoms are first and add any suggestions about their cause afterwards.

Diagnosing stress symptoms

'Symptoms' are any changes in your bodily or mental functioning that you find unpleasant and are different from how you normally feel. Try to describe them as accurately as possible and avoid jumping to the conclusion that they are due to stress. The doctor's primary role is to make a diagnosis, and this can only be done properly if all the relevant information is available. Even then, this may be difficult because many of the symptoms of stress can masquerade as other diseases that will have to be excluded from the frame.

This is because stress, as noted earlier, has effects on both the mind and body and symptoms that are entirely due to a form of mental stress can be completely indistinguishable from those caused by physical disease. If you put yourself in the doctor's shoes at this point, you can see the difficulty of the problem. 'This symptom – pain and spasm in the stomach area – appears to be a consequence of worry over possible redundancy, but I cannot be absolutely sure. What do I do? I could give some antispasmodics and something to reduce stomach acidity, then wait for the worry to subside, which I guess it will do once the job problem is sorted out one way or another.'

However, there is another scenario. The doctor, after ruminating a little, may act differently. 'It is just possible – I think at a level of risk of less than 1 in 100 – that these symptoms are the first sign of a serious disease, such as stomach cancer, gallstones or pancreatitis. If I fail to investigate this now, it may be too late to stop the underlying disease from becoming fatal and I could be considered negligent.' So, just to make absolutely sure, the patient is given an appointment with a specialist in bowel diseases to have tests done to exclude these diseases as causes of the symptoms.

This is entirely understandable and, in an age when the philosophy is 'someone to blame, make a claim', if investigations are delayed too long, the doctor could be successfully sued and this indeed could be completely justified (I have come across this in my own practice). The trouble is that for the 99 per cent who have a stress-related condition – the most common explanation of these symptoms being irritable bowel syndrome (discussed at length in two books in this series – Nicol, 1989 and 1991) – such tests are likely to lead to more psychological problems, those of hypochondriasis or health anxiety. The doctor may well explain that the problem is highly unlikely to be due to a serious disease, but the sufferer is still likely to worry that they have it. 'The doctor does not want to worry me', thinks the sufferer, 'but I would not be referred to a specialist for tests unless the doctor really thought something was wrong.' So, even if the investigations turn out to be negative – as they will much more often than not – it is natural for sufferers' thoughts to still trundle on in the same mindset – 'the doctor would not have referred me if there was nothing the matter, so they must have done the wrong tests. I will ask for more.' So you can see we have established a vicious circle, not a virtuous one, and it is hard work to break it (how this is done is described in Chapter 9).

Drug treatment

The most common mental health symptoms seen in general practice are those of depression or anxiety linked to stress. As noted earlier, these are collectively called 'adjustment disorders', but doctors hardly ever use this term (Casey, et al., 2001).

It takes a little time for a GP to unravel the tangled strands of adjustment disorders. It is much easier to identify a few symptoms, link them together and, hey presto, we have a mental disorder that can be explained to the patient in such a way as to increase the doctor's authority. So, in the past, the GP's explanation went something like this: 'I know that you are very shy and so whenever you have to get up in front of people at work and make a presentation, you are bound to be very anxious. I'm not sure what we can do about this apart from giving you a tranquillizer just before you have to get up and speak or, alternatively, enquire if you could move to a similar post where you do not have to make these presentations.' Now it has changed to, 'Your shyness used to be thought of as something that was part of living and you had to put up with. Now, we realize that it is a medical condition called social anxiety disorder. This is not your fault and research has shown that it is associated with a lack of a special substance, 5-hydroxytrypt-amine, or serotonin, in your nervous system. I will therefore give you a drug called fluoxetine (Prozac), which will put your serotonin back into balance.'

The second explanation is much more reassuring. Now the proper doctor is speaking. You are not quite sure what all these words mean, but they carry conviction and are clearly based on science. We will look again at the value of these explanations and treatments towards the end of this chapter. Before we do so, it is worthwhile trying to put yourself in the position of being a GP and seeing dozens of people every day with roughly similar problems. I emphasize the word 'roughly' here because, of course, to the individual sufferer from stress each of these problems is unique.

You may be at the end of your tether because a relationship is breaking down or you have just lost your job or one of your children is seriously ill or you have a court case pending – the list is endless. However, all of these are problems that have no instant solutions, otherwise you would not be sitting in the surgery. GPs cannot solve the problems or take them away and, rather than struggle to find a personal solution, it is so much easier to succumb to the blandishments of identification of conditions and treatments that follow naturally from these. So, apart from a few sensible words of advice, which are more likely to come if the doctor has a good background knowledge of your problems, there are very few options available that fit in to the average consultation period of seven minutes. It is only in old movies, and perhaps in private practice, that you will receive the proper amount of time necessary to ensure that the advice and help received is really tailor-made for your problem. Even then, this is often not achieved despite time being apparently unlimited.

The cry, 'I can't go on like this' is a plea for more than sympathy. Prolonged and severe mental stress becomes mental agony and cannot be tolerated. GPs have a way of reducing this degree of stress and making it more bearable. They can prescribe a drug or, more specifically, a 'psychoactive' drug – that is, one that acts on the mind. This group of drugs – tranquillizers and antidepressants – are prescribed more often than any other class of drug in medicine and it helps to know something about them. First of all, do they work? Are drugs successful in reducing the effects of stress?

The answer is 'yes' for most of the drugs of today, but often 'no' for the remedies of the past. The complicating factor is the 'placebo effect'. When a tablet or medicine is taken for any reason, there is often an immediate feeling of relief long before the medicine has had any opportunity to be absorbed into the body. This is because we believe that we have taken something to help us and the very act of believing makes us feel better. This effect is much greater if we have confidence in the person who has prescribed the medicine.

Many years ago, doctors had very little in the way of effective treatments. About the only common feature of medicines was that they tasted nasty and, according to Victorian logic, if something tasted unpleasant, it must be doing good. Most of these medicines, however, were placebos and the doctors who prescribed them often realized it. Those who did not often gave the drugs in higher doses and created new problems in the form of side-effects and sometimes these could be fatal. It is not surprising to learn that the science of homeopathy, in which toxic drugs were given in great dilution in order to stimulate the body to overcome the effects of disease, was introduced at this time.

Doctors also realized, though not always in a fully conscious way, that if they appeared to be highly knowledgeable men who seldom made mistakes and had a cure for every ill, they did far more good than if they appeared weak and ineffective. So, they developed their omnipotent airs and were always careful to keep a certain distance from their patients so the element of mystery was maintained. Looking back on this from a modern perspective you may feel that it was deceitful and unfair to act in this way, but if you talk to elderly people about their attitude to doctors, you will find that they often yearn for the old days when doctors were revered and could do no wrong. In fact, the doctors of today are much more effective than they ever were in the past, but close monitoring of their practice is relatively new and has been accelerated since the terrible case of Dr Harold Shipman, now identified as the greatest mass murderer in the United Kingdom. We would all like to think that in the past there were no Dr Shipmans anywhere in the world, but it is sad to reflect that, if there were, it is unlikely that they would have been detected.

Tranquillizers

Many of the tranquillizers of yesteryear were placebos and whether or not they helped people depended on the doctor's charm and personality. Of course, if placebos cured people or permanently helped to alleviate their symptoms, doctors would be happy to prescribe them all the time. However, unfortunately their effects seldom last longer than a few weeks. This may be quite satisfactory for some illnesses where the sufferers are going to get better anyway, but those of you who think you have harmful stress are likely to have had symptoms for much longer.

Alcohol

One of the original tranquillizers that was far from being a placebo was alcohol in all its forms. Alcohol is a powerful tranquillizer, although those who have never drunk to excess might find this hard to believe. A small amount of alcohol may feel like a stimulant, but this is an illusion, as it is really acting as a mild tranquillizer by first removing your inhibitions. In larger amounts, it calms you down and if too much is drunk you will become unconscious.

If you take alcohol for stress, it seems to work – at least at first. You stop worrying about whatever it was that made you worry, feel calm and relaxed and help yourself to another drink. The cycle has started, for one drink often leads to another in these circumstances. When the effects of the alcohol wear off, you are presented with the same problems that were there before you started drinking. So, it is only natural to drink again to return to that happy land of make-believe where stress is a five-letter word with no meaning. Unfortunately, alcohol is not just an escape from the problems of stress; it creates new ones and exacerbates those already present. The husband who does not get on with his wife and drowns his sorrows at the pub, the inefficient executive who removes his business worries at the bar of his club or the sportsman who fails to maintain his fitness yet boasts of his prowess in an alcoholic twilight world are all stereotypes from low-budget movies, yet they all exist. The downward path started by alcohol abuse is painfully obvious to everyone else but the victim, who will blame all except drink for his plight. People under stress who are already moderate drinkers are the most likely to find themselves moving down the slope towards alcohol abuse. The temptation to take just that little bit more alcohol is very strong and the excessive drinking pattern is established.

So alcohol is definitely out as a tranquillizer for combating stress, except in emergency situations when nothing else is available. What of the others?

Barbiturates

Barbiturates used to be popular tranquillizers, but they have exactly the same snags as alcohol and, in most countries, are no longer used except for particular members of the group used for the treatment of epilepsy. They tend to oversedate, impair judgement and are addictive when taken in regular doses. Some people can get away with taking them regularly at night for insomnia without becoming hooked, but those who take them during the day as well are almost bound to become addicted if they persist. As far as the brain is concerned, a barbiturate pill is the same as a large alcohol lozenge.

The only reason that there are many more alcohol addicts than barbiturate ones is that it is socially acceptable to drink alcohol, whereas barbiturates are available only on prescription from doctors and are rarely prescribed.

Benzodiazepines

The group of tranquillizers that are still prescribed is one that includes Librium (chlordiazepoxide), Valium (diazepam) and Mogadon (nitrazepam) (the trade names are conventionally given with capital letters and the generic name in lower case). These are all members of a group called the 'benzodiazepines'.

The reason your doctor will prefer these to the others is that they are much better at reducing anxiety and stress without seriously affecting other parts of the brain. Thus, they can reduce the impact of stress without greatly impairing judgement and coordination.

They are definitely not placebos. If you take a tablet, it takes about an hour to be absorbed into the bloodstream and then it begins to act. You feel calmer and more confident, but if you have taken too large a dose you will feel sleepy. Of course, if you are very nervous and only take a small dose you may notice nothing at all.

The effects of just one tablet last for about four hours. However, if you take them regularly, they can go on affecting you for over 24 hours. If you take one of these tablets regularly at night, it is bound to affect you the next day as there is no such thing as the perfect sleeping tablet that just lasts for the night and is completely out of your system by morning.

What will a prescription for one of these drugs do for stress? First of all, let us be clear what it will *not* do. It will not remove the stress or alter it in any constructive way. It is in no way a substitute for the personal decisions to combat stress that we described earlier and will come to again later in this book. It will not give you sudden insight into or understanding of the stress. People are getting to know more about the drugs they take and some of these statements may be obvious, but they are worth repeating. All a tranquillizer can do is take the edge off your reaction to the stress and relieve your suffering. In case the word 'suffering' sounds a little strong, let me emphasize that it can be a great deal worse. Torture is often a more apt description for the mental reaction to a stress that just grinds on interminably like a dentist's drill into the brain. If stress is producing this kind of reaction, it is ridiculous to deprive yourself of a tranquillizer because of strong principles that it is somehow wrong or a sign of weakness to take pills. By taking a pill when in this state, you can at least lessen the stress on your mind and body and at best allow yourself a breathing space, which helps you to decide on the best way to remove the stress.

Tranquillizers and dependence

It will be clear by now that if tranquillizers are being taken for stress they are best taken occasionally, at times when the stress becomes unbearable. If you take them regularly, there is a danger that you will take no further action to resolve the stress. You accept your lot as being not a happy one, but the taking of tranquillizers makes it tolerable. If you did not have them available, the unpleasantness of the stress might drive you to do something about it, something constructive that might eventually remove the stress altogether. It is difficult to get the balance right between emergency drug treatment and long-term psychological repair and adjustment. If you are in a state of paralysing anxiety, there is no more chance that you will work out a long-term solution to your stress than there is of winning first prize in a lottery, but, if you are cocooned in a cosy tranquillizer trap, you may delay taking the action necessary to move you forward. It is this dilemma that leads to the general recommendation that tranquillizer prescriptions should, in principle, be short term, generally for no longer than a few weeks.

However, there is another reason for not taking tranquillizers regularly. They can produce dependence and, rarely, addiction. This is not the same as addiction to alcohol or hard drugs, but you can still get hooked. If a first prescription was given for one or two weeks, to tide someone over a crisis, but was then repeated – not just once, but dozens of times – the tranquillizer that was originally like a crutch, to help you keep going while your emotions were repaired, becomes something you cannot live without. If the tablets were stopped for any reason, you would feel nervous and tense again and go back for another prescription.

The ideas in the preceding paragraph appeared in the first edition of this book in 1980 and showed the results of research that, at that time, had not yet been published but revealed that there was a significant problem of dependence with the benzodiazepine drugs (Tyrer, et al., 1981). We now understand a little more why this happens. If you take a tranquillizer for a short time, it stimulates a system in the brain called the GABA system. The stimulation of this system leads to a general calming effect and so stimulates the natural part of your body that is involved with calming down. Unfortunately, when you continue to take the tablets in the same dose for months or years, the natural GABA system says to itself, 'there's no need to keep working, someone else is doing the job for us', and so it goes to sleep. When the time comes to stop the tranquillizers, therefore, there is nothing to take over from the tablets and you have a major upsurge of anxiety, with panic, palpitations, sweating, dizziness, and feel as though you are having a withdrawal reaction. Of course you are, and when you take the tranquillizer again, it offers immediate relief.

Some of our personality types are more likely to have withdrawal reactions than others. The Gamma types have felt nervous all their lives and it is not surprising that they take to tranquillizers as a duck takes to water. Unfortunately, it is this group, together with the Etas, who have the most problems when they try to stop their drugs (Tyrer, et al., 1983). They go on taking the pills because all life is stressful for their constitutions and anything that reduces their nervousness is going to be in demand. However, it is much better to choose one of the techniques to reduce anxiety described in the last chapter because there are fewer problems with repeated yoga and relaxation training than with repeated swallowing of tranquillizers. The dependent Zetas have been guided to this chapter last because they, too, are more likely to become hooked than other personality types. Not only do they tend to rely on other people but also on medicines. Even if there is no need to go on taking them after the first prescription, they feel lost without them and demand more. It is even possible for them to become dependent on placebo pills in exactly the same way, so the problem is in the mind rather than in the pills. If you are either one of these personality types, be very careful about taking tranquillizers and certainly try to avoid taking them regularly.

There are many other tablets used to treat problems caused by mental stress and it is wrong to assume that they are all tranquillizers. There are stimulants and antidepressants and these act in quite a different way. Some are habit-forming and some are not, some work immediately, others have a delayed effect, some are dangerous when taken with other drugs and certain foods, others are quite safe. Just as doctors can give different tablets for diseases of different parts of the body, they can give different medicines for many mental reactions to stress, so do not assume that all tranquillizers are the same. Sometimes people are upset when they are given a tablet for nerves as they are convinced that it is their bodies alone that are reacting abnormally. If you have ever been in this position, you will know the feeling – you feel slighted because your evidence has apparently been considered unreliable and your judgement wrong. Although such feelings are understandable, they are unnecessary. We need to be reminded that the mind and body are not like separate countries, linked only by radio and telephone communication. They are more like close relatives, living and working together. Almost everything that influences the mind will also influence the body and vice versa.

So, a tranquillizer will not only reduce anxiety but also lower blood pressure a little (although if you have high blood pressure – hypertension – it will have little effect), lessen sweating and the pains of irritable bowel syndrome by relaxing the muscles in the gut. It tells the sympathetic nervous system and the other hormone regulators to slow down a little and the parasympathetic nervous system to stop slacking and come a little more into the picture. Temporarily, but only temporarily, it is bringing mind and body back to the balancing systems of healthy stress. However, if you sit back at this stage and do nothing further to correct the source of the stress, you will achieve very little and run the risk of dependence on the pills. This is a critical time in stress management. The pills have given you a breathing space, but they have not secured a solution. The ability to look at yourself in a more detached way should be the spur to finding long-term answers so you can look at your problems again in a new light and see a way ahead that was not clear before. If you use this opportunity wisely, you are likely to have no difficulty in stopping the tranquillizers when the time comes (provided that they are not barbiturates or alcohol).

Antidepressants

There are many ways in which your doctor can respond to your cry for help – I have only dealt with the most common ones here. Now that tranquillizers have been recognized as causing dependence, it is more common to be prescribed one of the newer antidepressants called 'selective serotonin reuptake inhibitors' (SSRIs), such as Prozac (fluoxetine), Seroxat or Paxil (paroxetine) or Cipramil (citalopram). These have been shown to reduce anxiety and stress as well as alleviate depression. They can even be helpful when no depression is present. However, do not be misled into thinking that there are no problems with withdrawing these drugs. These tablets can also lead to a form of dependence shown by unpleasant symptoms on withdrawal, but, until recently, these were politely called 'discontinuation effects' by the manufacturers. The outcome of all this is that, when reducing doses of any of these tablets, it is wise to do it slowly, tapering the dose to zero over a period of between two and six weeks in most instances.

At the beginning of this chapter, you will recall that I compared what the typical doctor used to and is now encouraged to say when giving Prozac for stress. By giving a clear diagnosis such as 'social anxiety disorder', emphasizing that it is a newly discovered condition (a classic case of old wine in newly labelled bottles), and muttering about serotonin deficiency, the case for giving Prozac is made much more eloquently than before. However, this is transparent nonsense as the real causes of anxiety, depression and stress are no nearer to and no further from being known than they were when Hans Selye published his paper in *Nature* in 1936. Maintaining that we have serotonin deficiency in our brains to justify the use of Prozac is no more scientific or true than saying we need to be bled by leeches because we have too much blood in our bodies.

Where to go from here

So, if you go to your doctor for help with stress, you should now know what to expect. The likeliest outcome is a prescription for a tablet or medicine (although this is a little less likely than it was a few years ago) and some reassurance. You are going to him in a crisis and being given first aid, but seldom more. If your GP knows you well, you may receive a great deal more than reassurance and be given helpful advice on combating your particular stress. Aspects of any physical disease may also be investigated or you may be referred for specialized psychiatric treatment. Although few of the treatments available to your GP are particularly good at relieving stress in the long run, they are useful in the very short term. Whether or not they will be of real value depends on how you use the breathing space the drug treatment gives you.

Doctors since the time of opium have had quick-fix treatments to reduce nervous tension, so if they choose not to give you such treatment it is because of its long-term dangers rather than incompetence or spite. The motto for the prescription of tranquillizers or antidepressants for stress is something along the lines of:

I'll give you this
Your woes will go overnight
But stop it soon
Or it may come back and bite.

The reason for different personalities reading this chapter early or late in the course of the book is related to this issue. The Alphas and Gammas read it early because they are less responsive to treatments described in other chapters and may need the help of drug treatment earlier in therapy. They also need to be reminded about the dangers of resorting to unofficial tranquillizers, such as alcohol, as a way of relieving their stress because these are much more dangerous than the prescribed kind.

Once the immediate pangs of stress have been relieved by medicines, the Alphas should move on to Chapter 10 and the Gammas to Chapter 9. It is impossible to predict when the move from what is, in effect, first aid to more fundamental treatments should take place because reactions to stress differ so much, but tranquillizers and antidepressants alone should seldom be taken for more than a few months. Nervous tension is relieved within hours or days, but it may take several weeks before depressive illness is brought under control. Once the first aid has worked, though, it is time for you to take over the responsibility for dealing with your stress again, not leave it in the hands of the doctor.

It is the people who regard medical treatment as the only way of coping with stress who are the ones to suffer most and some may stay on tablets unnecessarily. This would not matter if it solved their stressful problems, but it often makes them persist. The square peg remains in the round hole but sits a fraction more comfortably because it is lubricated by medicine. The desire to leave the round hole for a square one or convert your existing hole into a better shape gradually dies because of apathy and the stressed misfit persists.

Most of you will be moving on to other forms of treatment and can put the policy of personal responsibility for stress into effect. The Etas and Epsilons should go to Chapter 10 and the Deltas to Chapter 8. This leaves us with our placid Betas and dependent Zetas, who will be reading this chapter last. They do so for different reasons. The Betas, provided that they have been honest in completing their question-naires and are really placid types, will rarely get to the crisis stage of stress when a visit to the doctor is necessary. If they ever do, the stress has to be excessively severe, such as that endured by the naval rating on the battleship described at the beginning of this book. We are fortunate in peacetime that few stresses of this severity last long, so any drug treatment is only necessary for a very short period. I therefore feel quite confident that a single prescription would be enough. After this, the placid Beta's great resources of healthy stress would take over and the problem would be under control.

Our dependent Zetas have come to this chapter last because they are the most susceptible to discarding personal responsibility for stress. They have the tendency to hand over all the difficult problems of life to other people to solve and occupy themselves with the easy ones. They are only too happy to visit the doctor at the first sign of harmful stress because this will absolve them from doing something positive themselves to overcome it. It will also allow them to blame the doctor if the treatment is not successful. Dependent types are very good at making other people feel guilty for not trying hard enough and usually get more attention and concern than other folk. If tranquillizers or antidepressants are successful in making them feel better, they all too frequently sit back and think that there is nothing more to be done (apart from collecting repeat prescriptions regularly). Any chronic consumers of pills can make out that they are invalids and dependent types are better than most at this exercise. They are treated as though they are physically and mentally unfit and protected from many of the demands of life. However, in the long term, they will not do themselves any good and probably create more harmful stress in those around them.

Even if the doctor recognizes the dangers of drug therapy, there remain other problems. Zetas are not only likely to become dependent on pills, but also on people. They are among the persistent visitors to doctors' surgeries, whether or not they have any true illness. They can develop a strong relationship with their doctor that can spin out of control. The relationship is almost all one way – essentially selfish and quite unhealthy. Such patients forget that they are only one of many hundreds treated by their doctors and will often ask for advice about the most trivial problems and at the most unsocial hours. Abnormal dependence has to be dealt with in treatment, but I hope that Zetas will have tried other ways of overcoming stress first with therapists who have more time and special skills in turning stress to the advantage of treatment. I know this may sound harsh to those who are only a short way along the road to dependence, but if I have scared you off tranquillizers, it will have done some good.

8

Breaking bad habits

Harmful stress, as I emphasized earlier, is uncompensated stress. All the anti-stress devices are called into action, but fail to get the mind and body back into balance. We commonly assume that the stress goes on affecting us because of things happening around us and are reluctant to consider that we might be contributing to it in some way. In the last 20 years, it has been realized that the way we behave in response to stress has a great deal to do with its persistence. To use the jargon, we create feedback – that is, we positively reinforce stress in our attempts to control it. In more everyday language, we get into bad habits.

Breaking the bad habits of illness is really the province of psychologists because they are trained in the theory and practice of normal and abnormal behaviour. Psychologists, unlike psychiatrists, are not trained in medicine, and it is not always easy to seek their advice directly. It is possible, though, for doctors to refer people to psychologists if a problem is considered to be in their field. However, this chapter is concerned with advances in the treatment of harmful stress that have come from the research of psychologists and much of that is easily available.

Many forms of relaxation training have been devised by psychologists from first principles and we have already come across these in an earlier chapter. Relaxation training is a form of behaviour therapy. Although you may think it odd that feeling tense is a form of behaviour, if we consider its causes and effects in stress, it is very much a behaviour. When we feel tense, our muscles become tight and knotted and we cannot help noticing how different they are from when we are relaxed. The feeling of tension is unpleasant and often distracts us from other things that we should be doing. Like the nagging pain of a toothache, it reminds us that all is not well and, naturally, this makes us feel a little anxious. When we feel anxious, though, there is an increase in blood flow to the muscles, so the tension increases. Our positive feedback cycle has started. Each time we worry about our muscular tension, it gets worse, so there is more worry and still more tension. Relaxation training (and similar techniques) breaks into this cycle and, if successful, prevents it from getting out of control. It replaces the harmful cycle with a new one, the negative feedback of healthy stress. If we are able to make our muscles relax at will, whenever we feel tense, the cycle of muscle relaxation, then mental relaxation, then further muscle relaxation is developed.

Behaviour depends on feedback of many different kinds. If we do something and are rewarded for it, we are more likely to repeat that behaviour than if we are punished. Although we tend to accept this for parts of behaviour that involve our whole beings, we have been less inclined to accept it for parts of the body. However, psychologists have taken this further. They have suggested that even the activities of the autonomic nervous system can be regarded as behaviour that can be brought under conscious control. Autonomic systems are, by definition, self-regulating and so the idea that we can control the actions of our parasympathetic and sympathetic nervous systems is a revolutionary one. Although it has not been confirmed, it has led to an interesting new treatment for stress called 'biofeedback'.

Biofeedback

If you have looked into ways of treating stress, you have probably heard of biofeedback because it is widely advertised as being able to do just that. Many of the advertisements are misleading because they give the impression that stress can be measured on an instrument and you can tell your level of stress by checking the instrument reading. Nothing in the world of stress is as simple as that and to understand biofeedback we need to know the theory behind it. It is based on the idea that all the bodily reactions to stress described in Chapter 2 are potentially under our own control, provided we use the right techniques. Once they are brought under control, the positive feedback cycle we have just described with muscle tension is broken and harmful stress eliminated. The techniques of yoga and relaxation we talked about earlier also have the same aim, but they concentrate mainly on the mental side of the cycle. Where biofeedback differs is that, with the aid of special instruments, you can get a much better idea of how your body is reacting to stress than if you just rely on your senses. With this extra information, you can learn to control your body more effectively.

Let us look at an example. You will recall from earlier that when we become anxious, we sweat more than usual, particularly on the palms of our hands and soles of our feet. The amount we sweat can be measured by an instrument that records how much resistance there is in the skin to the passage of a small electrical current. When we sweat we produce a salty solution that lowers the resistance; when our skin is dry the resistance is raised. The instrument is called a 'psychogalvanometer' – it sounds more impressive than a sweat recorder. The level of resistance can be shown on a dial or converted into a noise. This is biofeedback. The 'bio' part means that the instrument measures a biological function and the 'feedback' part we already know about.

None of this is of value to us unless we can reduce how much we sweat in response to the feedback given. There is reasonable evidence that this can be done, although not everyone can do it really well. It would be too complicated to go into all the arguments for and against controlling simple biological functions by biofeedback, but, let us assume for the time being that we can. Does this mean that there should be psychogalvanometers in every chemist's shop and department store so that passers-by can be given an instant stress reading? When we feel stress is harming us, should we buy a personal psychogalvanometer to learn how to bring our sweating under control? No. The simple idea that because we sweat more when we are under increased stress, therefore sweating measures stress is wrong. First of all, there are many other reasons for sweating – stress is just one. When the weather is hot and humid, we sweat more and after vigorous exercise we also sweat profusely. This does not mean that we all get nervous when we exercise or else the Olympic Games would become the Panic Games and Inuits would never get anxious. The second reason is even more damaging to this idea. If we compared the amount of sweating in 100 people under stress with that in 100 calm people, we would find, on average, more sweating in the stressed group, but there would also be many individuals in the stressed group sweated less than the sweatiest people in the calm group. I am sure this fits in with your own experience. You must know at least a few placid sweaty people and a few nervous ones with dry skin. A dry-skinned nervous person under very severe stress will record a low stress reading on a psychogalvanometer and even if that person does not reduce the stress successfully, the reading will stay low.

The only people who may find biofeedback with a psychogalvanometer helpful are those whose sweating is closely linked to their general reaction to stress, but these form a minority. Although psychogalvanometers are relatively cheap, it is not a wise investment to buy one before knowing whether or not you are in the small group who are likely to find it helpful.

There are other instruments available that measure the functioning of different parts of the body. All of them involve sticking metal discs or pads to the skin close to the part of the body concerned. Heart rate and muscle tension are most commonly measured and even brainwaves can be recorded and played back to the person using a microphone.

The people who seem to be helped most by biofeedback are those who show harmful stress as muscle tension and pains, headaches and migraine. Provided that the right group of muscles is chosen and that when they are relaxed the symptoms lessen, the technique can be most effective.

When practising biofeedback, the person concentrates on reducing tension in the muscles. If successful, the feedback, usually in the form of clicks or a continuous sound, lessens. Even a tiny reduction in tension can be picked up, so the person can work at a wide range of manoeuvres to find which is the best at reducing the symptoms.

You will recognize many similarities between biofeedback, yoga, t'ai chi and other forms of relaxation training. Biofeedback is like a Western equivalent of yoga. Both have the same aim – to reduce tension and promote inner tranquillity. However, whereas yoga and meditation rely on mystical incantations and instructions, biofeed-back relies on an idol of the Western world – a machine that tells us about quantity more than quality. One stems from religion, the other from science, but they share more than they like to admit. This does not mean that they are the same treatment in deceitful garbs as the exercising of muscle and mind control in yoga and t'ai chi are very different from biofeedback, but sometimes the outcomes can be the same.

Changing response patterns

Biofeedback is just one way to unlearn the bad habits of harmful stress and there may be others that are suitable for your particular problem. If you can say of your problem, 'I know what I ought to be doing but somehow cannot seem to do it right', then you could be stuck in a bad habit. The chances are that something you do to reduce the stress is increasing it and that a programme designed to unlearn this harmful response may get rid of the stress. The wrong response can vary from being overweight but eating more after an argument or a bad day because it makes you feel better to being nervous with unreasonable fears (phobias) and avoiding all the places that bring on the fears and thereby making them worse.

Examples could easily be found to fill a whole book, but most of them show the same pattern. Some way of coping is learned that seems to work immediately, but, in the long term, makes the problem worse. The trouble is that people are reluctant to give up the ways that seem to work in the short term because the alternative may temporarily make them feel worse. If you take an alcoholic drink whenever you feel tense, you will usually feel better afterwards, but when the effect of the alcohol has worn off it is a different story. At a more complex level, if you respond to an argument with your husband or wife by saying nothing for three days, it will certainly avoid further argument during that time, but could cause long-term damage to the marriage. The tendency for us to do those things that we are rewarded for and stop doing other things that produce no immediate benefit depends on laws of conditioning. Where a psychologist can help is by setting up new rewards and punishments to replace the ones that are failing to resolve the stress. So, the 'silent treatment' after an argument between husband and wife is replaced by an agreement for both parties to talk through the difficulties until they have been sorted out.

Many people find it hard to believe that this type of approach is of any value in treating stress. So much of it appears to be common sense, so why should a specialist's help be needed? Help would not be needed if our heads always ruled our hearts and we always did the rational, sensible thing, but we are often led by our emotions to do things that we seem powerless to prevent. I have asked the ambitious, worrying, fussy and suspicious personality types to read this chapter earlier than the others because these types are more likely to have been conditioned to behave in certain ways than other types. To put it another way, they are more likely than other people to have developed bad habits. Of course, the type of conditioning will vary tremendously from person to person. The ambitious types are heavily conditioned by success, so everything they do that leads to material success is encouraged, even if it destroys mind and body in the process. The psychologist can show that success can be obtained just as easily by delegating more work and spending less time on it, without the damaging punishment of stress. The worrying types are conditioned by fear. By trying to avoid anxiety in life, they find it everywhere and, eventually, it becomes part of them. Real fears are replaced by imagined ones – round every corner there is a tiger waiting to pounce. By teaching how to master anxiety using relaxation techniques, biofeedback and self-assertion, these types can improve their self-confidence and prevent their surroundings from dictating their actions. They will still be worriers, but will no longer be imprisoned by anxiety. Our fussy types are similar in some ways. They organize their lives along rigid tramlines and get put out by change that is in any way out of the ordinary. They become conditioned into thinking that no change can be for the better and continue along their well-worn grooves when everyone else has adapted long ago.

We all have to be prepared for rapid and unexpected changes in life. Our fussy types, surrounded by stability, often cope extremely badly with bereavement. If we have been very close to a relative or friend for many years and he or she dies suddenly, a tremendous readjustment is needed. We have to reconstruct our lives, but if the central pillar has been taken away it is difficult to stop the whole house falling down. Most of us get by with support from other relatives and friends, taking solace in religious beliefs or throwing ourselves wholeheartedly into something quite new. However, our fussy types with their set routines find this extremely difficult and often take to ruminating about the dead person and continuing their lives in exactly the same manner as before. The first stress of the bereavement has not been resolved, so, gradually it becomes harmful stress because the necessary rebuilding has not been done. With psychological help this pattern can be avoided, but, if it gets out of control, the stress will eventually surface as severe depressive illness.

Suspicious types are conditioned by mistrust and jealousy and need strong secure relationships. Give them a chink of suspicion to work on and they will prise it wide open. A casual remark about liking another person will be interpreted as an indication of a secret affair that has been going on for months or years. Unfortunately, once a pattern of mistrust has developed it is almost impossible to deal with it by means of reason alone. The more the innocent wife denies that she is having an affair, the stronger is the belief of her husband that she must be having one, for otherwise why would she deny it so vehemently? If she chooses to be offhand about it, the jealousy is still reinforced, for then she is accused of hiding something. The psychologist has to start on a completely new tack in such a case, teaching techniques that avoid rumination and anxiety and alleviate suspicion indirectly.

It is not always necessary to have special help to break bad habits. By reading this chapter, you may have identified some bad habits of your own and can see ways in which you can change them. Your problems and goals will still be the same, but you realize that you have not been successful in getting rid of the stress because of a persistently inappropriate way of responding to it. Even if you do not think that the way you always use to cope with the problem is wrong, it would do you no harm to try a different way next time. Bad habits do not disappear on their own. Things you do make them persist or remove them. Doing nothing at all will also allow the habits to die out in time, but it may take many months and the ambitious types for one will not be able to tolerate this. Deconditioning is better, but it needs a push of some kind to start the process. Changing bad habits that have gone on for years is like opening an old door. The first time it is opened, it creaks and shudders before yielding to the weight and the hinges need oiling, protesting with creaks and groans. The more the door is opened, though, the easier it is to move it until, before long, no special effort is needed. Look for those hidden doors in your life before deciding that all your habits are good ones.

Alphas should now move on to Chapter 10, Betas, Zetas and Etas to Chapter 7, and Gammas and Epsilons to Chapter 9. The carefree Deltas have finished, apart from the final chapter. They are the group least liable to develop bad habits, in the psychological sense, but are much more likely to have problems because they have no habits! An action only becomes a habit if it is repeated and Deltas, in their endless search for variety, will seldom do the same thing twice.

9

Let's talk about it

We all talk about problems, some much more than others. This chapter is concerned with talking as a form of treatment for harmful stress and, if you have followed the book in the right order, you will realize that talking treatments involve people who have skills that members of your family and close friends do not normally possess, but there are many exceptions. The talking treatments are called psychotherapies, which provoke quite different reactions depending on personality type.

Alphas, as we know, never have enough time to do the things that they would like to do, and talking is unnecessarily time-consuming for them. The idea of talking as a form of treatment is something that often annoys them intensely. If the talk is in the form of concise advice that can be easily and quickly understood, this is not too much of a problem, but talking vaguely about their difficulties in the hope of understanding them better is quite another matter. Alphas are reading this chapter last because psychotherapy is likely to make their hackles rise. If, however, everything else has failed, it is in their interests to look at it seriously.

Placid Betas are quite happy to talk about problems, provided that the talking makes few demands on them. They adopt the policy that all is going to turn out for the best and there is no point in rushing things, particularly if it involves effort. So, psychotherapy for them has to be superficial – they will not take kindly to deep, probing questions about their feelings and wishes that force them to think too much. However, for most of their problems, a more superficial approach is ideal as the harmful stress Betas experience is not likely to last long.

Our worrying Gammas are sympathetic to any treatment that is going to stop them worrying. As they have been anxious all their lives, they have plenty of time so this is no object. Above all, they would like to know why they are so nervous and whether or not there is some deep-rooted cause in the long-distant past. They will take psychotherapy very seriously and cooperate well with the therapist. Delta types are also happy to talk about solving the problems of stress. They usually talk easily and well, but find more difficulty in persevering with treatment. Their need for variety makes them search for rapid solutions rather than follow a steady course taking up to several months. However, if they are prepared to stay the course, they can be helped, which is why they are reading this chapter at an early stage.

Suspicious Epsilons are in two minds about psychotherapy. They often need to discuss their difficulties, but they do not like disclosing confidential details about themselves. They will only talk openly when they have complete trust in the therapist. They are also highly sensitive people and do not take criticism well, so discussing ways in which to overcome stress requires patience and tact as well as understanding. The uncertain Zetas have no problems in talking, however. They positively relish the opportunity, but, although they often feel that they will make great progress and find the answers to their problems, all too often their doubts and uncertainties resurface. It is as though they are playing an interminable game of snakes and ladders in which they never get to the top of the board, sliding down a slithery snake just when they are within sight of their goal.

Fussy Etas share the concern of their fellow Alphas about the value of talk. They are quite happy with simple, straightforward advice, but do not like the vagueness of talk unless it is clear which goal it is being directed at. Although they say that they dislike talk because it does not lead anywhere, sometimes they are concerned because they feel threatened. Each Eta has a heavily fortified defence surrounding 'castle me' and always fears that camouflaged spies may enter through the back door when least expected. Order in life, with clear rules, preferably laid down by some external directive that can be followed to the letter, is the best form of protection. Letting people talk freely about personal subjects leaves Etas vulnerable. In place of order, there might be chaos and uncertainty, and the castle could come tumbling down. Attention to security is the favoured activity of the insecure and loose talk, even if it is meant in good faith, promotes insecurity. Making inroads into these defences is difficult, but may be worth the effort, and one advantage of being an Eta is that, once engaged, each will stick at the task until it is done.

I am not going to pretend that your reaction to talking treatment is necessarily going to fit in with the one given for your personality type, but you can at least see the wide range of reactions there are to psychotherapy. Up to now, we have only discussed talking in general terms. How can it counteract harmful stress and who should be involved in it? Psychotherapy can be carried out at several different levels. We all use it at its simplest level. Reassuring and comforting people in distress and listening to and commenting on their problems sympathetically are good examples. This can be done without any special understanding or great knowledge of the person in distress. At a deeper level of psychotherapy, we need to know something more about the sufferer. What sort of person is he or she and what special circumstances have caused this reaction at this time? In answering these questions, it is as though a surface map is made of the person and surroundings, a map that is unique but shares many features with others. The therapist should have special knowledge of the type of problem so that he or she can give constructive advice, advice that the sufferer is unlikely to have received from elsewhere. For this type of psychotherapy, it is important to go to the right person. If harmful stress occurs in a marriage, it is reasonable to consult a marriage guidance counsellor. Such counsellors are specially trained in understanding and advising about marital problems – they know from experience the features that make personalities clash and prevent difficulties from being resolved. As a result, they are not advising in a vacuum – they have seen problems like these before and can see solutions to them even if those involved cannot. If a marital stress problem is sexual, such as impotence, frigidity or premature ejaculation, further help may be needed, possibly from psychological treatments described earlier, and sex therapy is now an established discipline within the spectrum of psychological treatments.

If the harmful stress is related to problems of guilt or with life making no sense and having no meaning, then, depending on your religious convictions, the church may be the place to go for your psychotherapy. It may sound strange to say this, but a great deal of psychotherapy is involved in religion and talking with someone who shares your beliefs can be very helpful. The minister or priest has special knowledge of you and your type of problem and can point the way to a solution. The confession of sin is a most potent form of therapy and is, in fact, imitated by doctors practising psychotherapy. Wiping the slate clean and starting afresh is an excellent way to deal with harmful stress.

If the stress is bound up with the circumstances of day-to-day living, it may be appropriate to seek the help of voluntary agencies and social service departments. Although many think of social workers as just giving advice about housing and social security problems or rescuing those who are homeless, they also have skills in psychotherapy and are now part of multidisciplinary teams – that is, they have close working relationships with nurses, psychologists and other health professionals. They can also be invaluable in determining what benefits people are entitled to. So, in addition to practical advice, you may be involved in more fundamental discussions. We often bring problems on ourselves and, unfortunately, all too frequently we repeat our mistakes when the same circumstances arise in the future, blaming 'the system' or something or someone else for lack of understanding. Do not get angry, therefore, if this is pointed out during discussions. If you have tried over and over again to solve a problem and are going nowhere, at least consider the possibility that you may have tackled it in completely the wrong way.

The deeper levels of psychotherapy are usually practised by psychiatrists and psychoanalysts. They regard their task as being quite different from that of other talking treatments. They are not concerned with constructing a surface map of the person and problem, but a complete map, including all the deeper layers as well as what is shown on the surface. It is not easy to get to these deeper levels. Therapists probe them by analysing dreams and using other techniques, all of which involve talking – not just for a few minutes, but often for hundreds of hours. The common stereotype of a psychiatrist is that of a mysterious man who talks in a mid-European accent, seldom gives a straight answer to a straight question and carries out all treatment sessions with his patient lying on a couch. If you expect your psychiatrist to be like this you will almost certainly be disappointed, but psychoanalysis is based on this general approach. It is very difficult to recommend when to turn to this type of therapy because it is usually expensive and very time-consuming and the surface appearance of the problem often tells us very little of what is going on underneath. In general, it is better to consider the psychoanalytical approach only when the harmful stress has become chronic and has resisted all other efforts to remove it – and even then only if you are prepared to invest a great deal of time (and usually money, too) in finding understanding, if not always an answer.

Cognitive behaviour therapy

Cognitive behaviour therapy – and its predecessor, rational emotive therapy – is a psychological approach that attempts to alter thinking. This should not be thought of as mind-altering treatment or brainwashing, activities carried out under cover as it were, that attempt to wrest control from your own psyche and transfer it to someone else. Cognitive therapy asks the person being treated to re-examine their own thinking, find out if any aspects are unhelpful and may possibly be adding to the stress instead of reducing it, then make adjustments that lead to relief. The therapist travels alongside as this process is undertaken, asking questions, clarifying issues and sometimes giving greater understanding of reactions and feelings. The original treatment known as rational emotive therapy was, as its name implies, a set of approaches to bring emotion – which can sometimes be thought of as having a life of its own – within the framework of thinking and reason. This approach, pioneered by Tim Aaron Beck in the United States, has been shown in dozens of treatment studies to be at least as, and sometimes more, effective than most other treatments for depression, anxiety, hypochondriasis, self-harming behaviour, some forms of severe mental illness such as schizophrenia and bipolar disorder, as well as stress-induced disorders.

When cognitive therapy – sometimes loosely called 'positive thinking' – was first introduced, it was felt by many to be unnecessary. Of course the woman crippled with anxiety had fearful thoughts and the man with depression was convinced that he was useless because such thoughts naturally follow these emotions and it is the emotional disorders that should be treated. However, when you consider some of these thoughts, they are clearly wrong-headed. The person suffering acute attacks of panic, for example, is often convinced that he or she is going mad. Indeed, it is one of the fundamental fears in panic and is accompanied by the fear of losing control. However, people do not become mad (psychotic) in a panic attack and a gentle reminder that this is one fear that need not be entertained can be of value. Having some acquaintance with those who are viewed by others as mad also brings home the differences and can reinforce the feelings of sanity. Edward Elgar, the celebrated composer, often used to remind people when he was thought to be acting strangely, 'don't worry about me. I know all about this as I used to be in a mad-house'. Indeed he was as his first post was as a bandmaster at the County Asylum in Worcestershire, which was a major formative experience in his choice of career.

Cognitive behaviour therapy does not have to be given by a therapist in person – it can be given in the form of a book or other written material (in which case it is called bibliotherapy). Many of the successful books in the Sheldon Press series, such as those by

Paul Hauck and Windy Dryden (see the Further reading section at the end of the book), constitute cognitive therapy in the form of bibliotherapy. These may be studied to understand the principles and process of such therapy, so I will only give one example here.

A climber on a walking holiday is caught in thick mist on a long climb of 15 miles. As he comes off the summit of the last mountain, he misses his footing, falls over and twists his ankle. He still has four miles to travel before he reaches his base. He stops, makes a bandage out of two handkerchiefs tied together to prevent the ankle swelling and limps on. The ankle swells and becomes more painful, so he has to stop several times before he gets back to base, including once at a stream where the ice-cold water soothed his swollen ankle and helped to reduce the swelling. When he gets back, two hours after the injury, his mates are impressed by his fortitude and, when they see his ankle, they are surprised how well he has done. They think it would be unwise for him to continue climbing with them, but, after one day resting, he joins them again and is able to maintain the pace of others on the climb. He achieves new respect in the eyes of the others by the end of the holiday.

Contrast this with a similar injury in a different circumstance.

A young man is in a hurry to get to an appointment at an office in a city. He dislikes his job and wants a change. He is already late and irritably tries to rush past slow-moving queues of people. In so doing, he trips over a loose paving slab and falls, twisting his ankle. He rolls over in pain and passers-by are alarmed by his reaction, so, with his permission, telephone for an ambulance as an emergency. As he waits for the ambulance, he telephones the office he was rushing to, explaining his predicament, and they are very under-standing about his not being able to keep the appointment (even though he would have been late no matter how fast he had overtaken the queues of people, they do not know that). He is taken to hospital ten minutes later as an emergency. An X-ray shows that there are no bones broken, but examination clearly shows damage to the ligaments of the ankle and a bandage is applied. He feels unhappy bearing his full weight on the ankle and is given crutches at the time of discharge from hospital. He does not return to work for two weeks and sues the council responsible for the loose slab for his injury. This takes many months to resolve and is eventually settled out of court for a relatively small sum. A year later he feels he has still not fully recovered from the injury, has lost his job because he has taken so much time off work and is very angry towards the council for creating such suffering in his life.

What are the reasons for the differences between the two reactions to a similar injury? The first seems to have made a virtue out of his injury, his bravery has been reinforced by the reactions of his colleagues and the injury has had virtually no negative impact. In fact, he can almost be described as having benefited from it. This is sometimes known as 'steeling' – that is, the toughening of character that occurs as a consequence of adversity.

The second man seems to have crumbled in the face of similar adversity, even though it happened in much more favourable circumstances. The accident seems to have completely destabilized him and he is now functioning badly in most parts of his life. The injury seems to have acted as a trigger and sensitized him to illness.

Of course, if you have absorbed the information about personality types given so far in this book, you could argue that these differences can be explained by the first person being an Alpha and the second a Gamma, but there is more to it than that. The thinking and attitudes of the two men could not be more different. The first, despite being in a potentially threatening environment, is in control of his destiny and thinks of ways in which to overcome the handicap with the minimum of adverse consequences. The second is quite clearly not in control of his destiny. Like a raft on a stormy sea he is tossed hither and thither yet blames everyone else but himself for his problems.

How can cognitive therapy change matters? Let us look in on a treatment session with the second young man – Dave – to find out. See my comments in brackets, which give an explanation of what might be going on.

Therapist: 'Clearly you are still very upset by the accident – it seems to have got you down.'

Dave: 'Yes. I still feel so annoyed with the council. It was all their fault and they've got away with it almost scot-free.'

Therapist: 'OK. I know you think that it's all their fault, but perhaps we could just see if there are other explanations, in the same way that we have looked at this before. [This refers to the approach of examining any strongly held, apparently counterproductive, thoughts from another angle.] We can accept that the council should not have allowed paving stones to be insecure, but you told me earlier that the one you tripped over had been loose for many months, so why was it that nobody else had fallen over it?'

Dave: 'Just luck, I suppose. I always seem to be jinxed.'

Therapist: 'Well, was there anything you were doing on that day that was different?' [The therapist is getting Dave to go back and examine the accident from other perspectives, but, in a collaborative spirit, so that it does not come across as contradicting Dave's account.]

Dave: 'Well, I was in a hurry. I was always in a hurry with that job – so much pressure.'

Therapist: 'So, if you hadn't been in so much of a hurry you might not have fallen over the stone. Why was it that you were under so much pressure?'

Dave: 'Well, there were always so many deadlines.'

Therapist: 'Yes, but on that day had you been asked in an emergency to go to the office?'

Dave: 'No. I always went there on a Thursday morning. [Dave is beginning to get the point.] I know what you're getting at. You're saying that it's all my fault and if I was looking where I was going it wouldn't have happened. You're just like that council barrister who made me look a fool in court.'

Therapist: 'No, not at all. I'm just trying to understand how you were on that day. [Of course he's not like that nasty barrister, who was trying to win the case for his client in the typical adversarial way lawyers have. He's trying to help Dave to find other explanations.] Why was it you were so late?'

Dave: 'Well, to tell the truth, I didn't like the job at all and it was a struggle at times to get up in the mornings. I never really liked the job anyway – it was just the money that kept me going.' [Understanding is glimmering ever so slightly.]

Therapist: 'So, if you had been happier in the job you might not have been late on that day and wouldn't have tripped over that stone?'

Dave: 'You could say that, but the stone shouldn't have been loose.' [He's not quite ready to move off this line yet.]

Therapist: 'But this is interesting, because it looks as though the accident had one indirect advantage. Although you lost your job as a consequence it was not a job you really wanted anyway. What would have suited you more?'

Dave: 'I don't know. I just want something that pays the same amount of money.'

Therapist: 'Yes, but if we forget about the money for a second. If you really wanted to choose a job that suited you, what would it be?' [Dave has a second fixed thought to go with the council being responsible for his troubles – money is the most important part of work, which is a thought that many others have, too.]

Dave: 'Well, when I was at school, I did a lot of acting, but it would never do as a career. There's no money in it.'

Therapist: 'Never mind about that now. [This subject is worth coming back to – is there no such thing as a successful actor who is financially solvent? – but there are other things to pursue.] Were you happy when you were acting?'

Dave: 'Yes. There's that repertory theatre in the High Street. They're always trying to get me to go back and do some work for them, but, as I said, there's no money in it.' [Back to the fixed thought again.]

Therapist: 'Well, you've got a bit of free time on your hands at the moment. Why not pop down there before our next appointment and see if you can help out. Then let me know what happened. Write it down if you can. That can be your homework before I see you in two weeks.' [I know 'homework' is an irritating word that is a reminder of school, but the idea of asking Dave to keep a record of what happens – and particularly to write down his feelings immediately after an event – means that a more spontaneous and accurate record is obtained. If he did not do this he might well enjoy himself at the theatre but convince himself before the next appointment that his original view was right and then the potential for change is reduced.]

I hope you can see from this account what cognitive behaviour therapy is trying to do. It both attempts to change inappropriate thinking and move forwards to more appropriate corrective action. It is not an easy task to shift some of the fixed thoughts that are not helping, but doing it in a collaborative way generally avoids conflict and moves the agenda away from old to new thinking strategies.

One obvious question comes up at this point. If psychological treatments can alter our thinking and emotions, can they also alter our personalities? This is an important question and the best answer is unsatisfactory in some respects – 'personalities that are fully formed are relatively impervious to change, but those that are still uncertain and developing are susceptible to adjustment and change'. Most of the 'uncertain' group come under the heading of flamboyant or dramatic personality disorders and also tend to improve with increasing age, whereas the other types have a tendency to become more pronounced as they get older (Seivewright, et al., 2002).

So, it looks as though there are unlikely to be dramatic results from cognitive therapy with regard to personality change, but it is not out of the question. There is some encouraging work (Kate Davidson, 2000) that is beginning to suggest cognitive therapy can be of value.

What talking can and can't do for you

Approach the talking treatments for stress with a sense of realism. In the past, far too many people looked at psychotherapy as a magical journey into the depths of their unconscious where they would find the gremlin that had caused their troubles and which, when exposed and destroyed, would explain and alter everything. Dazzling insights into ourselves can happen, but they rarely change our basic personalities. What they are able to do – and this is where psychotherapy in all its forms can help – is strip off the layers of phoney personality that we all cover ourselves with from time to time. We protect ourselves to some extent with a coating or façade and often it is so impressive that it appears real. It deceives others so well that we also begin to think that it is true. If we fool ourselves in this way without realizing it, we are apt to become what we are not, parodies of ourselves in roles that others would like us to play but which are not our true selves. When you see people about you who seem to have undergone a transformation in personality, there is unlikely to have been any basic change. They have either peeled off their counterfeit façades or climbed behind new ones, but eventually the real personality will show through again.

So, please stick with your personality types as we continue the journey, unless you feel that you were being less than honest when you filled in the questionnaire. Deltas, Gammas and Zetas should now proceed to Chapter 10, Betas to Chapter 8, and Epsilons to Chapter 7. Alphas and Etas have completed their tour and now need only to read the final chapter.

10
Keeping fit

People have odd notions about keeping fit. Many think that they are fit if they feel well and have no signs of ill health, but, if asked to run to the end of the street they will be unable to get halfway there. They protest that to be a successful runner you need to be super-fit, which requires special training and should not be expected of the average person. Others think of fitness as the muscular strength of the body beautiful, and try to mimic Charles Atlas, Arnold Schwarzenegger and Mr Universe by strenuous body-building exercises and pumping iron. Yet others think that the only people who can achieve physical fitness are professional, full-time sportspeople and it is pointless for part-timers to get involved.

Exercise and its effects

What has fitness got to do with harmful stress? To answer this we come back to the idea of balance between mind and body. I noted earlier that we live in an era of specialization. Society forces us into spending much of our time using only the skills for which we have been trained. Because of increasing automation, very few of these skills involve healthy exercise. Even farm workers and manual labourers, who do far more healthy exercise in the course of their work than the rest of us, have many machines to do the jobs that their predecessors were forced to do with their bare hands. The rest of us are denied even a modicum of exercise in our work. We sit at desks in offices exercising no part of our bodies below the neck, so it is not surprising that these parts cry out for activity and fall into disrepair and disease if it is not received. We abuse our bodies still more with many of our habits. Breathing the polluted air around people smoking cigarettes or that in congested cities and industrial plants damages our lungs and makes us less able to meet the demands of exercise. We still eat too much of the wrong foods, stuffing ourselves with fats and carbohydrates rather than extra protein. The carbohydrates in sweet and starchy foods are excellent for giving us a rapid energy boost, but if we do not exercise our bodies, it is converted into fat, expanding the waistline.

97

It is all too easy in these days of refined and concentrated foods to eat more than the 2,500 calories a day that most of us rarely need to stay in equilibrium. If we consume more than this, we become fat and find exercising even more of a bind. Overweight people can be sluggish and need fewer calories than thin ones, so they find it harder than most to lose weight. All too frequently, they give up and decide that they are 'naturally' overweight and point to some distant relative who was huge, yet was hale and hearty and died at an advanced age.

The trouble is that when our bodies run to seed in this way, we have very few reserves to call on when our systems are put under stress. When discussing conscious healthy stress earlier in this book, I noted that when our sympathetic nervous systems are stimulated, we put our bodies and minds temporarily out of balance and the fitter we are the more rapidly we return to normal. For those who are unfit, it may take a whole day to shake off the effects, but there can be even worse results. An overweight man with furred-up arteries (atherosclerosis) and an inefficient heart has so little in reserve that even the excitement of watching a comedy show or sport on television can prove to be too demanding, with fatal consequences.

Keeping fit not only protects us from stress damaging our bodies but also aids our mental mechanisms. Sitting in a chair all day may appear to be physically relaxing, but it is actually a marvellous promoter of tension. All of us get frustrated and angry from time to time – Alpha and Delta types more than others – but we have to suppress the natural physical consequences of these feelings. We cannot club our colleagues over the head when they upset us or run into the distance when our boss approaches with a threatening scowl. However, if we can get rid of these frustrations later, such as by hitting a punchball vigorously while imagining that it is just the same size, shape and has as much sense as that annoying colleague's head or going for a long run or bike ride, we shall feel better and much more relaxed.

So, keeping fit both protects us from future stress and helps us to cope with current stress. The best way to keep fit is to exercise the whole body so that all parts build up reserves and become more efficient. Exercise in the form of running, swimming, walking or cycling is therefore a great deal better than weight-lifting, press-ups and all forms of exercise that take place while standing still. Such exercise also causes the release by the brain of pleasure-producing and pain-relieving hormones called endorphins, which are similar in many ways to heroin and morphine, but much safer. Now you can understand why some people are apparently 'addicted' to exercise.

Being fit is not necessarily related to muscle-building activities – those who choose the latter are usually more interested in vanity than health anyway. Really well-trained fit people are rarely muscular in appearance, although they have a higher proportion of muscle to other tissues than unfit people. Because there is very little or no excess fat, fit athletes may even be described as scrawny or weedy, but do not be put off by their appearance for there are tremendous reserves stored behind their lean frames.

Exercise and personality

What is the best way to keep fit? There is no best way for everybody – what you choose will depend on your personality type. The important thing is that whatever form of exercise you do, it should involve your whole body and be intense enough to increase your heart rate and make you a little breathless. By doing this you are training your body to be more efficient so that the next time you do the same exercise, you will be less breathless and recover more rapidly.

Alpha types have little time for physical fitness, but they are good at responding to a challenge. They like to be able to measure progress in exact terms, not just in the way they feel. It is best for them to set aside a defined period each day from their busy timetables in order to take their exercise. It should have a goal, something that can be bettered with increasing fitness. A points system following a competitive strategy with accumulation of points for good performance is ideal for Alphas. The system can be used for running, stationary running, swimming, cycling, walking and sports such as squash and basketball. This includes programmes for reaching and maintaining fitness. It will also help Alphas if they cut down on undesirable habits that handicap fitness. The stresses that they seek out in their lives make them more likely than others to be smokers, although thankfully this is much less common now than formerly. They will soon realize that their fitness programme is much easier to attain if they cut down their smoking or stop altogether. Once the tar is cleared out of their lungs, they will have no desire to return to the habit.

Beta types hate the idea of fitness programmes. With their

99

naturally placid temperaments, they cannot see any point in doing unnecessary exercise to get fit and they would not have the persistence to follow a points system. They are best advised to take their exercise in a more practical way. Their natural laziness inclines them to take the easiest way out of any problem and they rely too much on machines to do work for them. However, if they live only a short distance from their place of work, they can easily walk instead of taking the car. Better still, they can cycle, which is a marvellous way of keeping fit. Instead of using the motor mower on the lawn, they can root out that old hand mower that has not been used for years. Of course, it takes more effort, but the results are much more satisfying. Most of these changes will take a little longer than the lazy alternatives, but, as Betas are not too concerned about time, this should not be a problem.

Betas also tend to run to fat as they enjoy their food and are less active than other types. The chief reason I have asked Betas to read this chapter at an early stage is that sloth and overeating are the habits that are most likely to cause harmful stress in them. If they are overweight and increase their level of exercise, they are tempted to think that nothing more is necessary. However, exercise has to be long and strenuous to result in the loss of even some weight, so a diet will probably be needed as well. There are countless dieting techniques and I am not going to go into detail about any of them, except to say that, in medicine, when we find that there are hundreds of remedies for a condition, it usually means that none of them work.

Almost without exception, our Beta couch potatoes require a drastic reduction in the amount of carbohydrate in the diet. All the successful diets, if followed properly, lead to the body being temporarily starved of food. When this happens, the body's own stores of fat will be mobilized to make energy. Obviously during this process you are going to feel hungry, even ravenous. The temptation to nibble between meals or slightly exceed the diet quota becomes very strong. If you succumb to it, you may not lose weight, but, if you are honest with yourself, you should conclude it is not the diet but you who has failed.

Nervous Gammas often question the suggestion that physical fitness is going to help their problems as theirs are mainly mental. They have forgotten those times in the past when they had just finished some long or vigorous exercise, whether in sport or another recreation such as fell walking, rambling or even digging the garden. The feeling of relaxation that follows is not just the absence of tension in the hard-worked muscles, but a mental peace that sweeps over and replaces the worries of the day. Strangely, good exercise can be an excellent tranquillizer (remember those endorphins) and makes you healthier into the bargain. Just think what a relief it must be for the bodies of Gamma types to be healthily exercised. Their sympathetic nervous systems are always being stimulated for action – like runners on their blocks waiting for the starter's pistol to fire – but, far too often, they fail to act, paralysed in painful anticipation of the next stress to appear. If you are a Gamma type and cannot relax when you use techniques such as yoga and autohypnosis, try them again after a period of exercise such as running or swimming. You will find them to be much more effective.

Carefree Deltas need to do a range of exercises rather than concentrate on one and improve their performance of that alone. Their need for variety leads them into unusual hobbies and these often give scope for exercise. Again, the same points apply. If the exercise is sufficiently strenuous to produce some breathlessness and increase the heart rate, it is valuable and healthy, whether it is achieved by cycling penny-farthings, underwater swimming with breathing apparatus or abseiling down cliffs. There is a tendency for Delta types to drink more alcohol than other types and, if this becomes excessive, it will not help their physical fitness. If you take a close look at the regular drinkers at your local pub, how many of them do you think could run a mile without feeling shattered? Drink has a gradual effect on fitness and this takes place long before it does permanent damage to the stomach and liver. There is another message for the sexual athletes that so many Deltas perceive themselves to be: alcohol doesn't increase sexual performance, it reduces it – indeed, it is one of the most common causes of impotence.

Epsilons and Zetas have opposing personalities and need to take different forms of exercise. Epsilons are naturally solitary and prefer to exercise alone, so cross-country running is ideal. It allows them to take on the world alone. Such runners love the sport because it is for the individual; they owe nothing to others and are really more in competition with themselves than with others. Zetas are gregarious and need people, and their exercise is much more pleasant when carried out in groups. Jogging in particular can be a group enterprise. The strain of competitive running is absent and the pace is such that the whole family can take part. Sports that involve groups, such as doubles for tennis and squash, are also liked by Zetas. There is time to talk between points and playing in a team takes away the personal responsibility of playing alone. Solitary exercise is not worth exploring for Zetas – it has too many disadvantages to be taken seriously and, as we already know, they hate being alone.

Etas are fussy and methodical and, like most of their life's activities, exercise is taken seriously. It needs planning and organization and will usually be incorporated into a ritual. This will vary from person to person, but, once it has become established, it sticks. A run before breakfast, a walk with the dog in the evening, a swim every Tuesday and Thursday, a game of handball or squash every Friday, are just a few examples. Others may make fun of these rituals, but Etas are much better at maintaining fitness because of them. The important thing is to make sure that at least one exercise ritual is included in the repertoire.

Alphas, Betas and Etas should now move on to Chapter 9, Deltas to Chapter 7 and Zetas to Chapter 8. Gammas and Epsilons have now completed their tortuous route and can finish by reading the last chapter. Whatever the nature of their stress and personalities, I hope that all types now realize the value of positive physical fitness – as opposed to simply an absence of ill health – in adjusting to, overcoming and preventing the effects of harmful stress.

11

Closure

If you have followed the instructions in the earlier chapters – or even if you have not and my attempt to plot a 'personality-based trail' for you has simply irritated you – in this last chapter, all readers are together again. I have nervously headed this 'closure'. The reason I say 'nervously' is that I am not quite sure what the word means, but I have always liked the sound of it. This word is often used by psychotherapists when referring to the resolution of an episode of conflict and stress, so gives quite a different impression from the shorter word 'close'. Closure implies that the issue of concern, whatever it was, is now nicely sorted out and no longer a problem – the festering nest of vipers has now been replaced with a neat package tied up in ribbons that can be displayed with confidence whenever necessary. Of course, if it is no longer a problem it may not need to be displayed, so, while 'disclosure' is an open admission of something that attempts may have been made to conceal, 'closure' can be regarded as the confident concealment of something that can be produced whenever necessary, but is no longer regarded as important.

I would like to feel that this is what you are aiming for with regard to coping with stress. Unless I have failed quite lamentably in my arguments in the previous chapters, it is clear that it is impossible to avoid stress in the course of our lives and, indeed, attempting to avoid stress is the least effective way of coping with it. Adjusting to stress is the successful strategy to follow and, as each of us is different, this adjustment has to be a personal one. Hold on a minute, though! Whenever I read statements that emphasize our uniqueness, I realize that each one allows the writer to have a universal cop-out clause that justifies every outcome – 'I told you so, you can't predict anything in this business.'

In this book I have illustrated the importance of our personalities in coping with stress, but know that it is only one of many factors that influence how we deal with it. There are dozens of others – the length and severity of the stressful experience, whether it shows in mental or physical symptoms, whether it follows from problems in relationships or from external events and whether its resolution appears to be under our control or at the mercy of the gods. These are just a few.

I will return to the issue of personality. Each of us has an ideal level of stress that we regard as optimal. Below this level, we are bored and above it we feel under strain. It is clear from the rest of this book that my argument for making personality such a big issue depends on whether or not you agree that different personalities have different optimal levels of stress. I hope you do. Driving Alphas have the highest levels and Betas the lowest, Gammas and Epsilons have moderately low levels, Zetas and Etas moderately high ones, and Deltas a little higher still. These are not necessarily the levels of stress that they encounter in their daily lives and Gammas in particular would like their stress levels to be much less. These ideal levels indicate the amount of change in their lives and surroundings that each personality group would settle for in the absence of any other considerations. So, you can see that, without too much disagreement, it is impossible to choose a situation that would be equally stressful, or equally stressless, for all groups of people. The aim is to try and fashion an environment, a set of relationships, an occupation, a lifestyle, that is as near to the optimal level of stress for you as possible.

It is worthwhile following up the implications of this. There are now thousands of self-help books, videos, cassettes and other technological aids aimed at helping you to overcome stress and other problems in life. These give the impression that we are all on a common quest and have the same goals. Of course this is far from true and, even though some may feel that certain wishes are universal, such as a big win on the lottery, you would probably be surprised to hear that some people do not indulge in buying lottery tickets because they fear the stress – I use this word in its proper context – of a large win.

Nidotherapy

So, a large part of overcoming stress is to recognize who and what you are, and to fit you into this world in the best possible way. Such an exercise even has a formal name, which is 'nest therapy', or, 'nidotherapy' (see the Further reading section at the end of this book). This therapy is used when a mental disorder (or physical one) becomes intractable, stuck, persistent, permanent, immutable (choose any of these adjectives but they all mean the same in this context) and there appears to be nothing more that can be done.

However, it is wrong to give up at this stage as, if you cannot change the disorder, you can try to make the environment it has to fit into a more appropriate home.

This is where the nest comes in. A bird's nest seems to be a fairly simple, primitive piece of technology, but, like many glories of the natural world, it is a magnificent invention. The great thing about this bunch of old sticks, some hair, feathers and dried leaves is that it is flexible. It changes its shape to suit whatever is resting in it. Not many other beds are so snug and helpful. So, just as the poor reed warbler who has the misfortune to have a cuckoo laying an egg in her little nest hardly notices the difference when the baby cuckoo is born, neither does the nest. When the egg hatches, the fast-growing cuckoo turfs out the baby reed warbler chicks when nobody is looking and the nest adjusts perfectly to the big chick sitting alone and expanding fast. Nobody notices the difference and, even though Mrs Reed Warbler almost disappears down the gaping mouth of her apparent offspring when she feeds it, the fundamental good fit of mother, child and home remains completely intact.

Nidotherapy attempts to do the same for us. So, if a 'cuckoo' has come into your life and seems to have taken over, the same process of adjustment needs to be made. The fundamental aim of nidotherapy is to make the environment fit the problem rather than the usual one of altering the problem so that it achieves a better fit with the environment.

Could the questionnaire be wrong?

If you feel that the type of personality you were said to be as a result of your scores on the questionnaire was quite wrong, then you may doubt the rest of the advice that I have given. I can understand your feelings and agree that it would be silly to assume that the questionnaire is right and you are wrong. A personality questionnaire is only a screen, not a diagnostic prescription. We all have a mixture of personality features and only a few have one dominant characteristic that shows in all aspects of their lives. If your highest score on the questionnaire was only a few points different from those for the others, then no one personality feature is dominant and you have an even mixture that comes within the normal range. A maximum score of 25 or more (or 9 or more using the single scoring system) suggests that you really have been given the appropriate personality type. If it disagrees with your own assessment, try asking someone else you know well enough to give a frank and honest opinion. You may be surprised at their answers. We all have ideas as to the people we would like to be, and it is all too easy for us to pretend that we have some or all of these features in our own personalities. Most of us would like to think that we have a good proportion of the placid Beta features in our personalities and very little of the solitary and suspicious Epsilon ones. If the results of the questionnaire tell you otherwise ask yourself whether or not you have admitted the existence of all the skeletons in your personality cupboard before you blame the questionnaire. This is important because it can be a great help in deciding on the cause of a particular stress. For example, if you feel dissatisfied and mentally tense for no apparent reason as everything in your life is settled and serene, the cause may be that you are basically an Alpha type who is understimulated. You may laugh at the suggestion that you are driving and ambitious because nothing you have done to date suggests these qualities, but there *is* a tiger inside you, waiting to get out when you give it the opportunity.

If your maximum score on the questionnaire was between 21 and 25 points (or 5 and 8 using the single scoring system), the personality type indicated by the score is probably the predominant one, but other features are also important. It is quite possible to achieve high scores indicating apparently contradictory types, such as Alpha and Beta or Zeta and Epsilon. In such a case, the overall personality is a fairly balanced one.

More serious problems

It is useful to also consider the issue of more serious problems occurring as a direct consequence of personality features, which are grouped together as personality disorders. Now, nobody likes to be thought of as having a personality disorder because it is a label viewed as a term of abuse. It is rather similar to having body odour. We mutter about people behind their backs so often that frank discussion of it is thought of as unseemly, and we tend to avoid contact with people who are judged to have BO. This notion about personality disorder has been reinforced heavily since the millennium in England and Wales (but not in Scotland, where it has been avoided), by the introduction of a new diagnosis – dangerous and severe personality disorder, often abbreviated to DSPD.

Whether or not the introduction of this new diagnosis has been helpful remains to be seen, but it has certainly not helped the image of personality disorder. This group of conditions has always carried with it the belief that it is untreatable as you cannot shake off your personality any more than you can shake off your shadow, and applying the diagnosis to a person implies that two extra, very sticky, labels have also been attached – 'difficult' and 'unlikeable'. Small wonder, therefore, that when you add the word 'dangerous' you have a very unpalatable brew. By contrast, the simple terms 'anxiety' and 'depression' seem to be much more attractive and wholesome.

I think this notion is wrong for several reasons. First, we now have good evidence from many quarters that personality is not something that can be divided neatly into 'normal' and 'disordered'. It is best looked at as a range between 'so completely and utterly normal it astounds me' and 'the most disordered person one could ever contemplate meeting in one's worst nightmare'. Almost all the population has mixtures of positive and negative personality attributes between these extremes. The conditions near the extremes are within the same groups that you have already identified from completing the questionnaire in Chapter 3. The main personality disorders are the antisocial or dissocial (the extremes of the Deltas), schizoid and schizotypal (the extension of the Epsilons), borderline (exaggerated form of the Zetas), the obsessional (a large version of the Etas) and the anxious (the Gammas multiplied about three times). Just as you have identified some of the main characteristics of your personality by completing the questionnaire, you could also be said to have identified some of the features of the equivalent personality disorder.

This is relevant to the second reason, which is why personality difficulties or disorders should not be stigmatized as being conditions with which we would never like to be associated. Studies of personality disorder in the general population show that they are extremely common, with 8 to 10 per cent of the population having such a condition – a great deal more than most might expect. All this means that around one in ten of the population have sufficient difficulties with the sorts of people they are that this leads to problems in life that they would not be likely to experience if they had different personalities. Sometimes the diagnosis may indicate that there is something wrong with the society in which the sufferers are living rather than there being any personal deficiencies. In our own research, we classify personalities along a five-point scale, so a comparison between someone who has 'personality 1' with another who has 'personality 2' becomes much less emotive than the current unsatisfactory terminology.

Some final thoughts

So, do not be afraid to admit that you have a personality type or that at times you suffer from stress. These are qualifications for membership of the whole human race and those who claim to be different are deluding themselves and others. Matching your personality to your circumstances in life is one of the best ways in which to cope with stress. I once worked with a doctor in an accident and emergency department who was very committed to his work but never seemed to be influenced much by the successes and tragedies that surrounded him. When I tackled him about his apparent insulation from the troubles of his work, he just reminded me that 'life is an incurable disease that always ends fatally' and smiled. I suppose this can be interpreted as 'seeing the big picture' and, certainly, getting your personality in this type of frame, by taking the long- rather than the short-term view, is a good strategy.

For others who have been troubled by harmful stress in the past but are now free and those who have yet to deal with its unpleasant features, I hope you can see the value of the phrase 'prevention is better than cure'. Although we have seen that stress is not a disease in itself, it lies behind many forms of illness and doctors agree that they are not very good at curing these illnesses. This does not mean that they cannot help, but curing means removing the problem entirely so that not even a mark is left. Harmful stress has a habit of making indelible marks that cannot be removed, so even partial removal involves a lot of effort. It is so much better to prevent harmful stress from developing in the first place. Again and again, we come back to the concept of balance, which is at the core of all healthy stress. If our autonomic nervous systems can keep balance so well, surely our conscious nervous systems should be able to do the same. The trouble is that the rules are almost too easy. We have heard them so often that we disregard them. We need to keep a balance between work and play, activity and rest, social contacts and isolation, emotions and intellect, and between noise and quiet and many other opposing forces. As we have seen, the points of balance vary from one to another, but must be present somewhere. No one is going to remain well without some physical activity and even the most isolated hermit needs some contact with fellow human beings.

One of the conclusions reached by our visitor from outer space at the beginning of this book was that stress was a scapegoat in our society. Unfortunately, I think that there is some truth in this, but, if we are aware of the danger, it can be eliminated. We live in an age in which an explanation is demanded for every happening and more and more answers are forthcoming. However, we shall never have all the answers and many things will remain unexplained. Rather than admit this, or continue to look for the answer, people put it all down to stress. As stress can change itself into any shape at will, it can obviously fit the demands of any situation, but, all too often, it is an explanation in a vacuum. I am sure that reading this book has shown the futility of blaming stress for unpleasant events, feelings or illnesses and then doing nothing further about it. The recognition of stress is the beginning of a solution to a problem, not the end, and, although the way towards a solution, like your route through this book, may be a tortuous one, it is worth the journey.

I finish this book with a simple rhyming verse. Although this is now unfashionable, it summarizes the message of this book better than my prose:

A curious beast is stress?
The form it takes we can but guess
Though its charging head may impress
Its wagging tail can cause distress
And its reduction we may bless
But if it goes we're in a mess
The clear message I must address
Not to challenge it more or less
But the notion in you caress
That the best route to happiness
Is to live in peace with stress.
To turn the lock you need a special key
Please understand your personality.

You now have the complete message. Organize your life to promote your personality's strengths and avoid the demon of harmful stress. Good luck on your journey and don't look back.

Further reading

Some of the books listed below are marked with an asterisk. This indicates that they are books used by the professionals and so can be a bit more difficult for non-professionals to follow, but a lot can be learned from them, so why not see if they can help you understand your situation better?

*Beck, A. T. (1976) *Cognitive Therapy and the Emotional Disorders*, International Universities Press, New York. (The original book about cognitive therapy and its application to the treatment of common mental disorders.)

*Casey P., Dowrick, C., and Wilkinson, G. (2001) 'Adjustment disorders: fault line in the psychiatric glossary', *British Journal of Psychiatry*, 179, pp. 479–81.

Crystal, D. (1995) *The Cambridge Encyclopaedia of the English Language*, Cambridge University Press, Cambridge.

*Davidson, K. (2000) *Cognitive Therapy for Personality Disorders*, Arnold, London. (One of the first books to explore the place of cognitive therapy in altering personality features.)

Dryden, W. (1994) *How to Cope When the Going Gets Tough*, Sheldon Press, London. (Cognitive therapy writ large, plus a lot of common sense.)

Dryden, W. (2000) *Overcoming Anxiety*, Sheldon Press, London. (Ditto.)

Hauck, P. (1979) *Depression*, Sheldon Press, London. (Persuasive way of getting out of the trough of depression by virtue of your own efforts.)

Hauck, P. (1980) *Calm Down*, Sheldon Press, London.

*Hawton, K., Salkovskis, P. M., Kirk, J., and Clark, D. M. (1989) *Cognitive Behaviour Therapy for Psychiatric Problems: A practical guide*, Oxford University Press, Oxford. (Good account of all the ways in which cognitive therapy can help a big range of problems.)

*Marks, I. M. (1999) 'Computer aids to mental health care', *Canadian Journal of Psychiatry*, 44, pp. 548–55. (A look into the future when a great deal of psychological treatment could be given via a computer screen instead of at a clinic.)

*Mayou, R. A., Ehlers, A., and Hobbs, M. (2000) 'Psychological debriefing for road traffic accidents', *British Journal of Psychiatry*, 176, pp. 589–93. (Shows that debriefing is ineffective for post-traumatic stress.)

Nicol, R. (1989) *Coping Successfully with Your Irritable Bowel*, Sheldon Press, London. (A good example of how stress affects one in three of the population at some time in their lives.)

Nicol, R. (1991) *The Irritable Bowel Stress Book*, Sheldon Press, London. (Tells you what it is and what you can do about it.)

Osborn, D. P. J., King, M. B., and Weir, M. (2002) 'Psychiatric health in a sexually transmitted infections clinic: effect on reattendance', *Journal of Psychosomatic Research*, 52, pp. 267–72. (Shows how stressful these clinics are.)

Rosenman, R. H., and Friedman, M. (1961) 'Association of specific behavior pattern in women with blood and cardiovascular findings', *Journal of the American Medical Association*, 24, pp. 1173–84. (First account of Type A and B personalities.)

Seivewright, H., Tyrer, P., Johnson, T. (2002) 'Change in personality status in neurotic disorders', *Lancet*, 359, pp. 2253–4. (Shows that, over a long time period (12 years), people's personalities change, some becoming less marked and others becoming more so.)

Selye, H. (1936) 'A syndrome produced by diverse nocuous agents', *Nature*, 138, p. 32. (Famous article putting stress in a biological context.)

Shephard, B. (2002) *A War of Nerves: Soldiers and psychiatrists 1914–1994*, Pimlico, London. (Excellent book showing the different forms of stress you can come across in battle – and there are many of them. Also helps to aid understanding of post-traumatic stress disorder.)

Tyrer, P. (1986) *How to Stop Taking Tranquillizers*, Sheldon Press, London. (What to do when you can't stop taking those wretched pills.)

Tyrer, P. (1999) *Anxiety: A multidisciplinary review*, Imperial College Press, London. (A book that I would like to think is not just for the professionals but may be difficult for others. It is a warts-and-all account of the mess anxiety has got itself into.)

Tyrer, P. (2002) 'Nidotherapy: A new approach to the treatment of personality disorder', *Acta Psychiatrica Scandinavica*, 105, pp. 469–71. (Account of the principles behind treating the environment, not the person.)

Tyrer, P., Owen, R., and Dawling, S. (1983) 'Gradual withdrawal of diazepam after long-term therapy', *Lancet*, 1, pp. 1402–6. (Study showing that tranquillizer withdrawal problems depended to a large extent on personality features.)

Tyrer, P., Rutherford, D., and Huggett, T. (1981) 'Benzodiazepine withdrawal symptoms and propranolol', *Lancet*, 1, pp. 520–22. (First trial showing that dependence and withdrawal symptoms occurred with tranquillizers from the benzodiazepine class.)

Zubek, J. P. (editor) (1969) *Sensory Deprivation: Fifteen years of research*, Appleton, New York. (Excellent summary of all those sensory deprivation experiments that some seem to have forgotten are a major creator of stress.)

Index